The Core of Masculinity

A Guide to Male Pelvic Floor Health and Vitality

Discover the Secret to Lifelong Intimate Health Through Simple, Proven and Targeted KEGEL Exercises

Evelyn J. Moritz

The Core of Masculinity: A Guide to Male Pelvic Floor Health and Vitality

Copyright© 2024 Evelyn J. Moritz
All rights reserved

For further information, please contact:

Evelyn J. Moritz

ejm.publications.info@gmail.com

Disclaimer

The information provided in this book is meant for informational and educational use only. It is not intended to replace guidance or care of a medical professional. If you believe you have symptoms mentioned in this book or any other illness, please consult with the appropriate health care professional for specific diagnosis and treatment. The author is not liable for the misuse or misinterpretation of the information provided in this book.

Sexual Health

Goes beyond

Physical Health...

Contents of the book

Introduction

Why Pelvic Floor Health Matters for Every Man?

When you think about masculinity, what comes to mind? Masculinity is often associated with attributes such as strength, power, vitality, confidence, and stamina in various aspects of life. However, a crucial component that often goes unnoticed is the pelvic floor. While pelvic floor exercises (Kegels) are commonly discussed in the context of women's health, particularly after childbirth, it is essential to recognize that men also possess a pelvic floor, which is just as vital to their overall well-being.

This book, "***The Core of Masculinity: A Guide to Male Pelvic Floor Health and Vitality***," aims to provide a comprehensive understanding of this crucial foundation of male health, confidence, and energy - your pelvic floor. You might be wondering, "What does the pelvic floor have to do with masculinity?" The answer: everything.

The pelvic floor plays a significant role in various aspects of masculinity. It is time to dispel the misconception that pelvic floor exercises are solely a "woman's thing." While men may readily discuss their physical achievements, such as bench press numbers or marathon times, the importance of pelvic floor exercises often remains overlooked or perceived as unfamiliar.

It is essential to shift this mindset and recognize the vital role the pelvic floor plays in maintaining male health, confidence, and overall well-being. The musculature extending from the pubic bone to the tailbone, akin to a supportive hammock, controls the urethral and rectal orifices, and sustains the base of the penis. These functions are pivotal to stronger erections, ejaculatory control, and overall sexual health. Regrettably, the importance of these muscles is often overlooked by the majority of men. Pelvic floor exercises are not commonly incorporated into fitness regimens or general health discussions, yet the advantages of strengthening the pelvic floor are essential and should not be disregarded.

This book serves as a practical guide to understanding and improving pelvic floor health, devoid of unnecessary medical jargon or overly technical details. It explores how strengthening these muscles can boost energy, enhance sexual performance, improve bladder and bowel control, and ultimately provide a greater sense of mastery over one's physicality and health.

Why Should Men Care About Pelvic Floor Health? The pelvic floor is a group of muscles that support the bladder, bowels, and sexual organs. These muscles are involved in everything from controlling urination to helping you maintain an erection. Most men do not consider the importance of these muscles until they experience issues. Like any other muscle group, the pelvic floor weakens over time if not properly maintained. Factors such as aging, a sedentary lifestyle, poor posture, or the neglect of targeted pelvic floor exercises can contribute to the weakening of these muscles. Weak pelvic floor muscles can lead to problems like erectile dysfunction, premature ejaculation and urinary incontinence, which can negatively impact one's self-confidence and quality of life. These are issues that no man wants to face. Fortunately, these issues can be addressed through the proactive strengthening of the pelvic floor muscles. In a world that often emphasizes external displays of strength like muscle mass, gym routines, workplace success, the importance of internal strength often gets overlooked. In many ways, your pelvic floor forms the foundation of your physical health. Emphasizing the importance of internal strength, a strong pelvic floor can enhance sexual function, boost core stability, and improve posture, which are crucial aspects of overall physical health. The individual's overall confidence is closely tied to their physical well-being. This internal fortitude is crucial for feeling assured and vibrant as a man.

As men age, the significance of pelvic floor health becomes increasingly apparent. While younger men may focus on the benefits of these exercises for sexual performance and strength, older men will find them essential for preserving independence and quality of life. The aging process often brings challenges such as urinary incontinence, fecal incontinence, recovery from prostate surgery, or erectile dysfunction. However, regular pelvic floor exercises can help mitigate these issues. These exercises are simple, can be performed at home, and do not require any special equipment. By investing a few minutes per day in your pelvic floor health, you can keep these muscles strong, enabling you to maintain control over your bladder, bowel, and sexual function well into your later years. Many men have experienced profound changes in their confidence and self-perception after taking charge of their pelvic floor health. By following the exercises and advice provided in this book, you will unlock your full potential, both physically and mentally. This book is designed to equip you with the necessary tools to effectively strengthen your pelvic floor in a straightforward and practical manner. It does not contain any extraneous content, but rather provides concise and applicable advice that can be immediately implemented. Each chapter meticulously examines key aspects of male pelvic floor health, encompassing basic anatomical knowledge, self-examination techniques, and step-by-step exercises (accompanied by illustrative drawings for enhanced understanding), as well as recommendations for seamlessly integrating these exercises into your daily routine. These exercises are simplistic, require no specialized equipment, and can be performed virtually anywhere. Many individuals have reported experiencing significant enhancements in their strength, control, and confidence within a matter of weeks. Pelvic floor health is not merely about mitigating issues such as incontinence or erectile dysfunction, but rather about optimizing overall well-being and quality of life. The benefits extend far beyond the immediate physical realm, positively impacting both your mental and physical well-being.

By the end of this publication, you will have acquired a robust understanding of the functionality of your pelvic floor muscles, their crucial importance, and, most importantly, effective methods for strengthening them. With a little bit of effort and consistency, you will witness improvements in your sexual health, core strength, and overall vitality. The journey to becoming the best version of yourself starts here— and it starts from within both physically and metaphorically. Are you prepared to harness the full capabilities of your pelvic musculature? Let's proceed accordingly.

Chapter 1: Understanding the Male Pelvic Floor

Understanding the Male Pelvic Floor

It's probably not the first thing that comes to mind when you think of fitness or health, but your pelvic floor is like the unrecognized hero of your body. The pelvic floor is an essential, yet often overlooked, component of overall physical well-being. While individuals may focus on developing visible musculatures, such as the biceps, abdominals, or gluteal muscle, the pelvic floor, hidden deep within the body, plays a crucial role in various essential bodily functions. This musculature is central to one's physical, sexual, and emotional performance. We don't notice these muscles until they stop functioning well. It is not until the pelvic floor weakens that individuals become aware of its importance, as the resulting symptoms, though initially subtle, can become disruptive and difficult to ignore. Many people accept these embarrassing symptoms as an inevitable consequence of life, without fully comprehending their underlying cause. Imagine your body as a house, the pelvic floor acts as the foundation, supporting everything from your spine to your organs. When it is strong, you feel stable, powerful, and in control. Conversely, when it's weak, things start to fall apart - a weakened pelvic floor can lead to issues such as sexual dysfunction or bladder problems. But here's the good news: it is important to note that, like any other muscle group, the pelvic floor can be trained and strengthened. Trust me, your body will thank you for it.

Sexual Health

does not exist

without

strong pelvic floor muscles!

Anatomy of the Pelvic Floor

Let's see where the perineal muscles are.

To perform pelvic floor (Kegel) exercises correctly, you first need to understand where your pelvic floor muscles are. Simply put, the perineum is the area of your body that sits on a bicycle seat—that is your pelvic floor. This "intimate part" of your body, these muscles, situated between the pubic bone at the front and the coccyx (tailbone) at the back, play a crucial role in regulating urination and defecation.

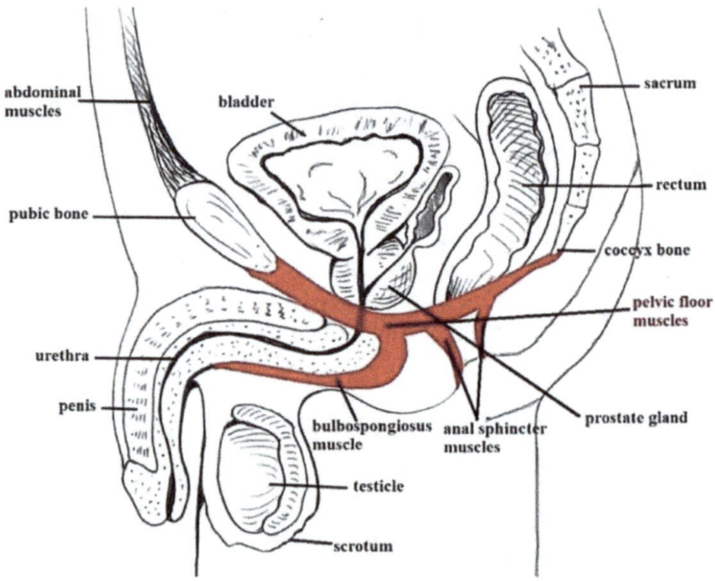

The pelvic floor can be envisioned as a taut hammock spanning the base of the pelvis, supporting the internal organs. For males, a well-functioning pelvic floor is essential for prostate health and sexual function. This hardworking, multitasking system of muscles, ligaments, and connective tissue provides both active and passive support to the pelvic organs. Despite the importance of these muscles, they are surprisingly small. Unlike the large muscles of your arms or legs, the pelvic floor muscles are tiny, with a surface area and thickness about the size of your palm. Yet, their influence on your body is enormous.

The pelvic floor comprises three distinct layers: the internal, middle, and external (also known as the superficial) layers. The primary muscles forming this "hammock-like" structure are collectively referred to as the **levator ani muscles**, which include the **pubococcygeus (PC)** muscle, the **iliococcygeus muscle**, as well as the **ischiocavernosus** and **bulbocavernosus muscles**. You don't need to memorize these names to understand their importance. The PC muscle serves as the "captain" of the pelvic floor muscles, responsible for contraction during sexual activity, supporting erections, and controlling ejaculation.

The ischiocavernosus and bulbocavernosus muscles play a supportive role by maintaining blood flow to the penis during an erection, which is essential for sexual stamina. During orgasm, the rhythmic contraction of the bulbocavernosus muscle, which encircles the corpus spongiosum (the structure in the penis that encloses the urethra), assists in the expulsion of semen (ejaculation). Robust pelvic floor muscles can significantly enhance sexual satisfaction for both the individual and their partner, which serves as a compelling motivational factor.

In the male anatomy, there are two openings in the pelvic floor: one for the urethra, allowing urine to pass from the bladder to the penis and exiting through the tip of the glans; and the other opening at the anus. The pelvic floor muscles firmly wrap around these openings to maintain their closure when necessary.

Imagine two circular muscles around both the anus and urethra: the **internal** and **external sphincter** muscles. The internal sphincter muscles, located in both the urethra and anus, are involuntary. They remain firmly closed unless the individual is actively urinating or defecating. These muscles are regulated by the **sympathetic nervous system**, which oversees the body's automatic functions. They relax and open only when the body triggers the urination or bowel movement reflex. In contrast, the **external sphincter muscles** are voluntary. This implies that individuals can consciously tighten them, providing additional closure when necessary, such as during moments of urgency, whether it is diarrhea or a sudden need to urinate. These muscles serve as a secondary layer of defense, offering extra control over these vital bodily functions. Both the internal and external sphincters completely encircle the urethra and anus, making them essential for managing bladder and bowel functions.

Pelvic Floor Dysfunction in Men

Dysfunction in the pelvic floor muscles is increasingly common among the male population. Sedentary lifestyles, chronic constipation and straining, aging, or even medical procedures such as radical prostatectomy can weaken these muscles. When the pelvic floor muscles are compromised, individuals may experience urinary incontinence, gas or fecal leakage, or even difficulties with erections. The perineal muscles in men are less sunken and more strained compared to those in women. The part of the superficial perineal muscles that surrounds the urethral and vaginal opening in females supports the base of the penis in males. Since the movement of these muscles is visually apparent in men, learning and voluntarily controlling pelvic floor exercises is often more straightforward. Although the structure of pelvic floor muscles is similar in both genders, differences in anatomy (due to variations in pelvic size and reproductive organs) influence their precise positioning and function. Nonetheless, in both men and women, these muscles are essential for maintaining proper bladder and bowel control, as well as overall sexual functioning. The male perineum is more protected than the female perineum, which is open and arranged to facilitate childbirth. These muscles are like the control panel of the pelvic region, constantly operating behind the scenes. However, similar to any control panel, when things go wrong, one can notice the problems quickly.

Fortunately, once an individual comprehends the functionality of the pelvic floor, they can undertake measures to strengthen and support it, thereby maintaining optimal long-term health.

What are the functions of the pelvic floor?

Now that we have established anatomy, let's talk about what these muscles actually do. The pelvic floor is essentially a silent, multitasking complex. Basically, it's like that friend who's always there for you, whether you realize it or not. In animals, due to their quadrupedal stance, the burden on the muscles that close the pelvis is minimal, as the weight of their internal organs is primarily supported by robust abdominal muscles. However, in humans, with the evolution of bipedal movement, this responsibility has shifted to the pelvic floor muscles.

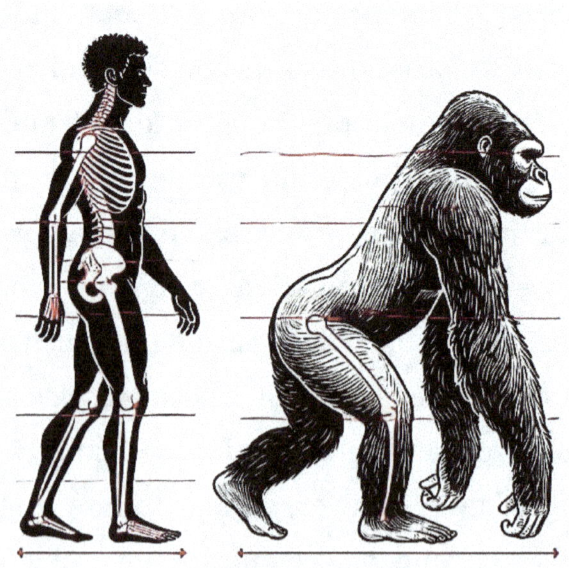

These muscles, which form a flexible "trampoline" at the base of the pelvis, hold the organs in place against the constant pull of gravity. Furthermore, this trampoline-like structure resists the pressure generated within the abdominal cavity, especially during activities such as lifting or straining.

The pelvic floor plays a crucial role in regulating the orifices that pass through it: the urethra and rectum, which connect to the external environment. The pelvic floor's primary function is to support the pelvic organs and control the pelvic exit. Its muscles are responsible for opening and closing the urethral and anal sphincters based on the body's physiological needs, whether during urination, defecation, or maintaining continence. For males, these same muscles also contribute to the angle and quality of an erection, as well as forceful ejaculations, influencing all sexual functions.

The pelvic floor contains two types of striated muscle fibers: fast-twitch and slow-twitch fibers. Fast-twitch fibers contract rapidly, generating intense, short-lived bursts of exertion, while slow-twitch fibers are responsible for prolonged, less intense muscle activity. This can be illustrated through an example. When one sneezes, the fast-twitch fibers in the pelvic floor contract suddenly to prevent urine leakage. Conversely, when the bladder is full, the slow-twitch fibers maintain continuous muscle tension to hold in the urine until urination takes place. When training the pelvic floor, it is essential to strengthen both types of muscle fibers to ensure full functionality in various situations. This comprehensive approach improves bladder control, sexual function, and overall core stability.

What Factors Contributing to the Weakening of the Pelvic Floor?

Why do pelvic floor muscles weaken? Several factors contribute to this, many of which are tied to the modern lifestyle. In human civilization, where individuals predominantly assume an **upright posture**, the pelvic floor muscles are constantly subjected to pressure. These muscles, once positioned perpendicularly, now adopt a nearly horizontal orientation due to our erect walking stance, bearing the weight of our internal organs. This shift can lead to physical complications, particularly if the pelvic floor muscles have been weakened or damaged by various factors. Such weakening often results in early symptoms, such as urinary incontinence, difficulty maintaining erectile function, or discomfort from hemorrhoids.

While **aging** is undoubtedly a contributing factor to the weakening of the pelvic floor, it is not the sole culprit. Many aspects of our modern, sedentary lifestyle, coupled with certain habits and health conditions, can progressively undermine the strength of this essential muscle group. This deterioration does not occur instantaneously but rather accumulates over time.

The **sedentary** nature of contemporary **lifestyles** plays a significant role in this process. Individuals now spend numerous hours in a seated position, compressing these delicate muscles from below. Furthermore, **poor postural habits**, such as slouching forward, can exacerbate the pressure exerted on the pelvic floor from above. Over time, these habits make it harder for the pelvic muscles to keep up with our daily demands.

Even basic daily tasks, such as using the bathroom, can contribute to pelvic floor issues. Many men strain unnecessarily during urination or defecation, employing improper techniques, (**forcing (rapid) urination**) instead of using methods that reduce stress on the bladder and pelvic muscles. Another significant risk factor is **straining during bowel movements**. Individuals may not realize that when they are exerting substantial abdominal pressure just to pass stool, they are also placing immense strain on their pelvic floor muscles. Over time, this can lead to serious damage.

Furthermore, **obesity** is a concern. Carrying excess weight, particularly more than 10 extra kilograms, applies additional stress on the lower abdominal organs. This extra load presses down on the pelvic floor muscles, overburdening them and making it more challenging for the muscles to function effectively.

Additionally, common **chronic respiratory diseases** or **allergies**, which involve **frequent coughing or sneezing**, are another unexpected contributing factor. When the body produces these strong, involuntary movements, the force shakes the pelvic organs and can cause strain on the muscles and ligaments that hold everything in place. When you cough, sneeze, or laugh, the abdominal pressure increases dramatically in your abdominal cavity, and if your pelvic floor muscles aren't strong enough, they won't be able to withstand the force. This could result in gradual urine leakage or a diminished sense of control over bodily functions. These repetitive, abdominal pressure-inducing situations can gradually weaken the pelvic floor, thereby increasing the risk of incontinence.

Chronic stress is another detrimental factor for the pelvic floor. When an individual experiences stress, the pelvic floor muscles tend to tighten, constricting blood vessels and limiting circulation. This deprives the pelvic floor muscles of the necessary nutrients and oxygen, hindering their proper functioning. **Smoking** exacerbates this issue, as nicotine is a potent vasoconstrictor, reducing blood flow to the perineal region. And let's not forget, smoking often leads to chronic coughing, which further burdens the pelvic floor.

Strenuous physical work and **improperly executed exercises**, particularly those involving heavy lifting without core support, pushing, or pulling, pose a risk as well. **Lifting**

heavy weights in the gym, carrying heavy objects, or lifting another person, if done without considering the sensitivity of the pelvic floor, can stretch and lengthen the supporting ligaments. While striving for improved health, one may not fully recognize the potential damage being done to the inner muscles. Increased intra-abdominal pressure can exert strain on the lower organs. Persistently engaging in such behaviors may result in unnoticed damage.

Frequent inflammation of the pelvic region, such as in prostatitis (inflammation of the prostate), can diminish the tone of the pelvic tissues involved, leading to a weakened pelvic floor.

Similarly, **weak or inflexible connective tissues**—whether due to genetics, aging, or hormonal changes—can leave the pelvic floor vulnerable to even minor stresses.

Any surgery affecting the pelvis minor or lower abdominal regions pose risks by potentially damaging nerves or muscles. **Nerve injuries**, in particular, can impair continence and sexual function.

And if you're someone who spends long hours sitting— whether at a desk or in a car, the lack of movement can cause **poor circulation and muscle fatigue in the pelvis**. When muscles aren't properly oxygenated, they become weaker and less capable of appropriately supporting the functioning of the pelvic floor muscles.

Even the **choice of apparel**, such as tight underwear or pants worn for extended periods without changing posture, can restrict blood flow to the pelvic region, decreasing oxygen supply and contributing to muscle strength decline. Only the muscle / organ adequately supplied with blood can work properly!

The effective functioning of the pelvic floor is essential. It is noteworthy that many of these risk factors do not operate in isolation. Issues with continence and pelvic floor dysfunction often arise when several of these factors combine or when the natural mechanisms of urination or bowel function become compromised. **Neurological conditions** such as multiple sclerosis or Parkinson's disease can frequently lead to direct pelvic floor problems, including muscle weakness, urinary incontinence, and sexual dysfunction. In certain instances, **specific medications** may trigger incontinence and erectile dysfunction (ED) as side effects. Most people don't realize how small these muscles are, though their impact on intimate health is massive. When considering the multitude of factors that can affect them, it is evident that numerous men are at risk. However, comprehending these risk factors is the initial step toward prevention. Fortunately, it is never too late to strengthen these muscles. Through heightened awareness, care, and exercises such as Kegels, one can protect and enhance their pelvic health, leading to long-lasting vitality and confidence.

Chapter 2: Men's Health Conditions Linked to a Weak Pelvic Floor

The Impact of Weak Pelvic Floor Muscles

Pelvic floor muscles may not be the first thing that comes to mind when thinking about men's health, but their importance is undeniable. These muscles constitute the foundation of the core, significantly impacting various aspects of physical well-being, including bladder control and sexual performance. This section of the book will explore the most common conditions associated with weakened pelvic floor muscles in men and demonstrate how proactive measures can substantially improve both health and quality of life.

Let me start with a **story** that might sound familiar. A personal acquaintance of mine, whom I shall refer to as Tom, used to scoff at the idea of pelvic floor exercises. "Kegels are for women," he'd say with a grin, dismissing it as irrelevant to manhood. Fast forward a few years, and Tom starts experiencing occasional urinary leakage, after going to the restroom. No big deal, right? Until one day, he laughed hard during a work meeting and—let's just say it wasn't only laughter escaping. That was his wake-up call to take pelvic floor health seriously. And now? Tom is the biggest advocate for pelvic floor exercises.

We've all had those "oh no" moments—the surprise sneeze, the uncontrollable laughter, or the unexpected jump that makes you feel a little less in control of your bladder than you'd like. While it is not exactly cocktail party conversation, it is more common than most men realize. And that's just the tip of the iceberg when it comes to the consequences associated with a weakened pelvic floor. The pelvic floor muscles support essential bodily functions, and they often deteriorate over time due to the constant pressure and strain they endure daily.

Let's dive into why every man should prioritize his pelvic health, the hidden costs of neglecting it, and the benefits that come with strengthening these key muscles. When the pelvic floor muscles are weak, the negative effects can be life-altering, as they support vital functions.

Stress Incontinence: When Urine Leaks at the Worst Time

You may not consider bladder control until it becomes a problem. Take **stress urinary incontinence (SUI)** for example. One of the first signs might be **involuntary urine leakage**. Have you ever had an unexpected trickle of urine when you sneeze, cough, or laugh a bit too hard? This is known as stress incontinence, and it can happen when the pelvic floor muscles, responsible for controlling the bladder, aren't doing their job effectively. While many men associate bladder leaks with older age, stress incontinence can affect men at various life stages, particularly after prostate surgery or due to chronic physical strain, which can be both embarrassing and frustrating. A more serious issue is **urge incontinence**, characterized by a sudden, uncontrollable urge to urinate, often resulting in leakage before reaching the restroom. Although common after prostate surgery, this condition also can affect men of all ages.

The Science Behind It: The bladder relies on a network of coordinated muscles and sphincters, working in harmony with the pelvic floor to hold and release urine as needed. If the pelvic floor is weakened, increased abdominal pressure from everyday activities like coughing, lifting, or laughing can cause small amounts of urine to leak out, as the muscles are unable to maintain the bladder's complete seal.

How to Address It: Fortunately, regular pelvic floor exercises can strengthen these muscles, reducing the likelihood of stress incontinence. By dedicating a few minutes daily to targeted exercises, such as Kegels, men can regain control over their bladder, preventing those embarrassing incidents.

Fecal Incontinence: The Lesser-Known Issue
Another common, yet less talked about, issue is **fecal incontinence**—the involuntary loss of stool or gas can be a distressing condition. It may arise due to surgical

procedures, the aging process, or even chronic constipation, and is often associated with weakened pelvic floor muscles. These pelvic muscles play a crucial role in regulating bowel movements by supporting the rectum and controlling the anal sphincter. In the absence of this support, it becomes challenging to maintain control over stool or gas, leading to unexpected and undesirable incidents. Weak pelvic muscles, combined with poor bowel habits, can also contribute to the development of **hemorrhoids**.

The Role of the Pelvic Floor: Just like with urine control, pelvic floor muscles play a key role in holding stool in place and releasing it at the appropriate time. When the pelvic muscles weaken, the anal sphincter may fail to close fully or retain stool until one are ready to use the restroom, resulting in accidental discharge. This issue can be particularly frustrating, as it not only affects physical comfort but also undermines self-confidence. Imagine being in a public place and suddenly realizing you have had a bowel accident. The emotional toll can be heavy.

What Can Be Done: Pelvic floor exercises, coupled with appropriate dietary choices, can provide substantial relief. Strengthening these muscles can restore control over bowel movements, ensuring fewer (if any) embarrassing episodes. Adopting a regular exercise regimen and increasing your dietary fiber intake can serve as a proactive measure against fecal incontinence.

Prostate Health: The Connection with Pelvic Muscles

The well-being of the prostate gland is central to men's overall health, particularly as they age. An often overlooked area, the pelvic floor supports the prostate and its functioning. The prostate already experiences reduced blood flow due to its location and the sedentary lifestyles many individuals lead. When the pelvic floor muscles do not function optimally, the prostate becomes more susceptible to infection and inflammation. Whether you are recovering from prostate surgery or managing a benign enlarged prostate, your pelvic floor muscles play a crucial role in your recovery and overall health.

Post-Surgical Recovery: For men who have undergone prostate surgery, especially for conditions like prostate cancer, one of the unfortunate side effects can be urinary incontinence. This occurs because the muscles supporting the bladder and urethra are disrupted during the surgical procedure. A weakened pelvic floor can delay your recovery and increase the likelihood of long-term incontinence.

How Pelvic Floor Exercises Help: Strengthening your pelvic floor before and after prostate surgery can significantly accelerate the recovery process. Studies have shown that men who practice pelvic floor exercises before surgery experience less post-operative urinary incontinence, while those who start post-surgery see faster improvements. These exercises ensure that the muscles remain strong and capable of supporting bladder function during this critical period.

Premature Ejaculation: Timing is Everything

Premature ejaculation (PE) is a prevalent sexual challenge faced by many men, though it is commonly underreported. There is no universally accepted timeframe for defining premature ejaculation, as it varies among individuals. Generally, PE is characterized by ejaculation occurring earlier than desired by the man or his partner, often before or shortly after penetration. While PE may be attributed to factors such as nervousness or excitement, in numerous cases, it can be attributed to weakened pelvic floor muscles. This condition affects men of all ages and can lead to sexual dissatisfaction for both partners. Imagine this: you are in an intense moment with your partner, and you feel like you are going to finish sooner than you would like. By engaging the pelvic floor muscles, individuals experiencing PE can effectively "pause" the ejaculation process, thereby extending the sexual experience.

How Pelvic Floor Strength Affects Ejaculation: During sexual activity, strong pelvic floor muscles help you control the timing of ejaculation. Pelvic floor muscles are directly involved in controlling the release of semen. Strengthening these muscles can significantly delay ejaculation, providing greater control and endurance during sexual intercourse.

Comprehending the sensations preceding ejaculation is also crucial in mastering control.

Learning to Control Premature Ejaculation: Premature ejaculation can be frustrating, but it's important to recognize that it is a manageable condition. The secret to addressing premature ejaculation lies in learning to contract and release the pelvic muscles during sexual activity. Regularly practicing Kegel exercises can provide greater control over these muscles, enabling the individual to delay ejaculation and prolong sexual pleasure for both themselves and their partner.

Erectile Dysfunction: The Hidden Cause of Erection Problems

Erectile dysfunction (ED) is often perceived as a circulatory issue, and while blood flow certainly plays a role, weak pelvic floor muscles can be a contributing factor. In many cases, men experience difficulties with erections not due to their cardiovascular health, but rather due to poor muscle control in the pelvic region. Maintaining a firm and lasting erection is not solely a matter of desire, but also a reflection of physical health, particularly the strength of the pelvic floor muscles. The pelvic floor muscles play a crucial role in erectile function by supporting the pelvic organs and regulating the blood flow to the penis. When these muscles contract, they help retain blood within the penis, sustaining an erection. However, if the muscles are weak, maintaining an erection becomes challenging.

The Pelvic Floor's Role in Erections: The pelvic floor muscles underpin the base of the penis and are integral to the process of achieving and maintaining an erection. Upon contraction, these muscles prevent blood from leaving the penis during an erection, ensuring firmness. Conversely, if the pelvic muscles are weak, this mechanism becomes less efficient, leading to difficulties in maintaining an erection. Sexual health is not solely about the physical ability to perform; it is also significantly influenced by mental well-being. Stress, anxiety, and fatigue can impair sexual performance, causing temporary erectile dysfunction (ED). When the mind is overwhelmed, the body's response is affected accordingly.

A Story About Pelvic Floor Exercises and Erectile Dysfunction

Here's another **story** example. Jack was in his 40s when he first started having **trouble with** his **erections**. Jack had always been in great shape, he ran marathons, lifted weights, and lived an active lifestyle. But suddenly, things in the bedroom weren't working like they used to. "It was embarrassing," he admitted. "I didn't know what was going on." Jack was initially unaware of the underlying cause of his condition. Upon further investigation, he determined that the issue stemmed from the weakness of his pelvic floor muscles. Consequently, he commenced performing Kegel exercises, which are commonly recommended for pregnant women. Although he felt ridiculous at first, he soon observed positive results from this regimen and his self-confidence returned. Jack's discovery highlights an important fact that all men should be cognizant of: pelvic floor exercises can be one of the most effective and natural methods to address erectile dysfunction (ED). Weak pelvic floor muscles may allow for the rapid drainage of blood from the penis, leading to the loss of erection.

Reclaiming Your Sexual Health: Fortunately, the pelvic floor, like any other muscle, can be trained and strengthened. By incorporating pelvic floor exercises into one's daily routine, these key muscles can be reinforced, thereby enhancing the ability to achieve and maintain erections. These exercises represent a natural, non-invasive approach to improving sexual health, making them a viable alternative or complement to pharmaceutical treatments such as Viagra. Pelvic floor exercises also can help bridge the gap between mental strain and physical performance by giving you greater control over sexual functioning.

Pelvic Floor Health Beyond the Bedroom

The state of one's pelvic floor health has a significant impact beyond the realm of sexual function. Pelvic floor musculature contributes to **core stability** and **overall postural** alignment. The pelvic floor works in tandem with the core muscles to maintain an upright posture, support the lower back, and prevent slouching. Over time, a weakened pelvic floor can lead to **chronic lower back pain** and poor posture, which affects not only one's physical well-being but also one's self-presentation and confidence. Preserving the health of these muscles is essential throughout the various stages of life.

The Benefits of Strengthening Your Pelvic Floor

The benefits of dedicating time to improving one's pelvic floor are numerous. They extend beyond simply avoiding issues, unlocking new possibilities for health, vitality, and self-assurance.

Better Bladder Control

One of the most immediate advantages of pelvic floor exercises is improved bladder control. A stronger pelvic floor enables the regaining of control over one's body. Individuals will no longer have to worry about sudden, uncomfortable, and often embarrassing leaks during strenuous activities such as heavy lifting, running, or jumping, granting them the confidence to fully enjoy life. Whether one is an athlete or simply wishes to maintain dignity as they age, the ability to control bladder function is a significant advantage. Furthermore, these exercises can enhance bowel control, helping to prevent urgency or minor accidents that can occur.

Better Posture and Core Stability

Many men focus on developing abdominal muscles for an aesthetically pleasing appearance, while neglecting deeper muscles, including the pelvic floor, which forms the foundation of the core. Core strength is not merely about aesthetics, but rather the stability and support the body requires for movement, balance, and strength. During physical activities, such as running or prolonged sitting, a robust pelvic floor functions discreetly behind the scenes to support your movements. Conversely, a weak pelvic floor may lead to poor posture, back pain, and reduced physical performance. Conversely, a strong pelvic floor helps stabilize the spine, enhancing the efficiency of movements and reducing the risk of injury and back pain, thereby enabling sustained physical activity. You will find it easier to maintain proper posture and balance, whether engaging in gym workouts, lifting heavy objects at home, or simply waiting in line at the grocery store. By incorporating pelvic floor exercises into your routine, you are not only improving your sexual health but also strengthening the core foundation of your body. A robust core not only looks appealing but it also feels good. In essence, a strong pelvic floor supports your masculinity from the inside out.

Preventative Health

Initiating pelvic floor exercises now helps mitigate many common issues men face later in life. It is far more effortless to maintain strong pelvic muscles than to rebuild them once they have weakened. By incorporating Kegel exercises into your routine, you are investing in your future health and well-being.

At Any Age: The Importance of Early Pelvic Floor Exercises

The Early Advantage

For younger men, commencing pelvic floor exercises at an early stage is crucial for establishing long-term health. These exercises are not exclusively intended for older individuals or those facing medical concerns. By incorporating pelvic floor exercises into your routine, you are laying the foundation for a life free from the preventable issues discussed previously, such as sexual dysfunction, urinary incontinence, and poor posture. Consider it akin to investing in a solid foundation for a house. One would not wait until the roof collapses to address the structural integrity, would they? Maintaining your pelvic floor early on is analogous to ensuring a stable foundation for the years ahead.

Mid-Life Matters

For men in their 40s, 50s, and beyond, the motivation to commence pelvic floor exercises becomes increasingly pressing. This is often the period when health concerns, such as prostate problems or declining testosterone levels, begin to impact bladder control and sexual performance. Strengthening the pelvic floor assists in counteracting these age-related changes and provides a natural means to preserve vitality, without relying solely on medications or other interventions.

Pelvic Floor and Sexual Health

Positive Impact on Libido: Supporting Sexual Confidence and Vitality

Libido isn't just a matter of desire, it's a combination of physical, emotional, and psychological factors. The psychological factors play a crucial role in an individual's physical readiness and sexual confidence. A healthy pelvic floor is essential in this regard. When one feels in command of their body, capable of managing erections, avoiding discomfort, and fully engaging in intimacy, their sexual confidence naturally increases. Weak pelvic floor muscles can adversely impact one's self-esteem, particularly if they lead to issues such as premature ejaculation or erectile dysfunction. Struggles with sexual performance often create a barrier in interpersonal relationships. Individuals may feel inadequate or embarrassed, leading them to avoid intimacy out of a fear of embarrassment rather than a lack of desire.

A robust pelvic floor can transform one's sexual experiences. Improved erections, longer-lasting performance, and more powerful orgasms are all linked to these muscles. During arousal and orgasm, the pelvic floor muscles contract rhythmically, heightening sensations and intensity. When these muscles are strong, the contractions are more powerful, resulting in more pleasurable sexual experiences. An additional benefit is greater control over ejaculation and enhanced erectile function. One will find that their stamina improves, and they can delay ejaculation for more extended periods, making intimacy more satisfying for both parties. As one enhances their muscle strength, they may also notice an increase in their sexual desire. The connection between physical capability and confidence, as well as libido, is evident. The advantage of pelvic floor exercises is that they can be performed anywhere, at any time, making them a convenient addition to one's daily wellness routine.

Enhanced Energy and Stamina

Surprisingly, working on the pelvic floor can also increase overall energy levels. By engaging these deep muscles, the core is strengthened, which in turn supports posture and physical balance. This stabilizing effect and increased energy means individuals will feel more robust and agile in their daily activities, whether at work, in the gym, or during intimate moments. This can be viewed as an enhancement of the internal strength system, helping to prevent injuries and providing more power in one's movements.

Just as in weightlifting or martial arts, mastering the smallest muscles often provides the greatest advantage. The pelvic floor acts as a hidden powerhouse; once accessed, it opens the door to greater stamina and vitality.

Conclusion

Regardless of age, pelvic floor exercises offer more than just physical strength; they also build confidence. When one has control over one's body, it is reflected in their posture, performance, and overall sense of well-being.

Unlocking a version of oneself that feels strong, vital, and prepared for future challenges is the objective. Confidence in professional, intimate, and personal realms commences with a positive self-perception, which pelvic floor health directly supports.

Attending to one's pelvic floor is not merely a passing health trend or a concern for later in life. It represents long-term, sustainable health and vitality. By concentrating on strengthening these muscles, individuals not only prevent common issues such as incontinence and sexual dysfunction but also enhance their confidence, energy levels, and overall well-being. Regardless of age, whether in one's 20s or 60s, it is never too early or too late to prioritize pelvic floor health. Now that the significance of pelvic floor health is understood, the next step is to learn how to effectively strengthen it. In the following chapters, practical exercises and routines will be explored, which can be easily incorporated into one's lifestyle to ensure the pelvic floor remains in optimal condition. So, let's commence the journey towards building a foundation for a healthier and more confident self.

The youthfulness of the perineum is independent of age!

Chapter 3: Learning Step-by-Step the Basis of Pelvic Floor (Kegel) Exercises

The Basics of Kegel Exercises

If you have made it this far, you have already discovered the secret superhero living within your pelvis: your pelvic floor muscles. The pelvic floor muscles, located within the pelvis, serve as a vital, yet often overlooked, component of the human body. For those who have recognized the significance of these muscles, an important step has been taken towards improving overall health and well-being. With a comprehensive understanding of the pelvic floor's anatomy and its crucial functions, one can now delve into the practical application of exercises designed to strengthen, increase the elasticity, and optimize the support provided by these muscles. These exercises, commonly referred to as Kegel exercises, are simplistic, discreet, and when performed correctly, can yield remarkable benefits, ranging from enhanced bladder control to improved sexual health. It is important to note that, similar to any exercise regimen, proper technique is of the utmost importance when executing Kegel exercises. To this end, it is essential to demystify the origins and definition of these exercises. The Kegel exercises were 'developed' (stolen) in the 1940s by Dr. Arnold Kegel, an American gynecologist, who sought to address the issue of urinary incontinence, particularly in women following childbirth. However, it is worth acknowledging that the foundation of these exercises can be traced back to the ancient practices of women in China and Thailand, who had been performing similar pelvic floor strengthening techniques for centuries without the specific nomenclature. The pelvic floor exercises have become the preferred treatment option for pelvic floor dysfunction. Although initially designed to assist women, these exercises have also been found to benefit men. The pelvic floor exercises can be considered a comprehensive full-body workout that can be performed at any time and location without the need for specialized equipment or gym membership.

The IWT® Difference: Why Intimate Wellness Training® Pelvic Floor Exercises Are Unique

The Intimate Wellness Training® (IWT®) methodology is distinctive in its holistic approach. In contrast to Kegel, the exercises of Intimate Wellness Training® (IWT®) are integrated, not only using simple muscle contractions, but combining them. Unlike traditional Kegel exercises, IWT® incorporates techniques to strengthen all types of pelvic floor muscles, including both fast-twitch and slow-twitch fibers. This is crucial as the fast fibers are responsible for quick, forceful contractions (such as preventing urine leakage when sneezing), while the slow fibers are responsible for sustained contractions (like holding in urine when the bladder is full). Furthermore, the IWT® approach focuses on preventing pelvic injuries by protecting the pelvic veins, which are particularly vulnerable in men suffering from conditions like hemorrhoids or varicocele. By training both types of muscle fibers and addressing overall pelvic health, the IWT® provides a more comprehensive and preventive approach to pelvic floor exercises.

Some Tips Before You Start to LEARN the Exercise Program

1. **Empty Your Bladder:** It's always best to start with an empty bladder.
2. **Set the Right Atmosphere:** Turn off your phone or put it in "Do Not Disturb" mode and avoid eating a heavy meal 1–2 hours before exercising. Wear comfortable, loose-fitting clothing and stay hydrated, but avoid drinking too much water right before starting.
3. **Use Props if Necessary:** If you have knee problems, place a soft cushion under your knees for extra comfort.
4. **Fingertip Test:** Unsure if you are contracting the right muscles? Place your fingertips on your

perineum (the area between the scrotum and anal opening) to feel the gentle squeeze when you contract.

5. **Relaxation is Key:** After each exercise, rehydrate yourself with enough water, and give your body time to relax.

6. **Be patient!** Do not proceed to the next exercise section, until you are not sure doing a movement /contraction correctly.

Are There Any Contraindications?

Kegel exercises are generally safe for most men, but there are a few scenarios where caution is necessary:

- **Pelvic Tumors:** There is some debate among doctors about whether physical exercise is safe for those with pelvic tumors. While some believe exercise could worsen the condition, others argue that proper blood circulation from exercise might help. Always consult your doctor first. Anyway, considering that proper organ function is largely dependent on adequate blood flow and oxygen supply, it's only logical to conclude that light physical exercise can significantly improve one's condition. Pelvic floor exercises, like Kegels, are no exception. These exercises not only strengthen the muscles but also promote better circulation throughout the pelvic region, enhancing the flow of oxygen-rich blood to the tissues. By regularly engaging in Kegel exercises, you are not just working on muscle strength, you are encouraging a healthy, well-oxygenated environment for your pelvic organs, ensuring they function optimally.

- **Catheter Use:** If you have a catheter, Kegels should be avoided until it's removed.

Exercises To Warming Up And To Make Conscious The Function Of The Perineal Muscles

Engaging in pelvic floor exercises may initially seem to be exploring an unfamiliar domain. It is uncommon to hear individuals at fitness facilities discussing the development of their pelvic floor musculature. However, mastering these muscles can bring about transformative benefits, not only for one's sexual well-being but also for core strength and overall vitality. This chapter will delve into the process of locating and exercising these muscles.

How to Develop Body Awareness to Control the Function of Your Muscles

The foundation for mastering pelvic floor exercises lies in cultivating body awareness and learning to effectively control one's muscles. A crucial aspect of this process is distinguishing the sensations between muscle contraction (strengthening) and relaxation. Both are equally essential in maintaining a healthy pelvic floor.

To assist in building this awareness, a series of exercises will be provided that not only teach the engagement and relaxation of pelvic floor muscles but also help you feel the subtle, imperceptible movements of these small yet pivotal muscles. Through practice, you will learn to refine their control, making it easier to perform pelvic floor exercises correctly and experience the full benefits.

How to Breathe and Relax During Kegels

During the performance of Kegel exercises, the coordination of one's breathing with the movement of the pelvic floor muscles can significantly enhance the effectiveness of the exercise. Proper breathing not only helps maintain control but also promotes relaxation, preventing unnecessary tension in the pelvic area.

As you contract the pelvic floor muscles, you should take a deep breath in through the nose. This should allow the abdomen to expand slightly as the lungs are filled completely. When the contraction is released, you should exhale slowly and fully through the mouth, allowing any tension to dissipate with the breath. This rhythmic flow of inhaling to engage and exhaling to release helps you remain mindful of both the contraction and relaxation phases, which are equally important for building strength and flexibility in the pelvic floor.

Relaxation is a crucial component of the process. After each contraction, you should take a moment to ensure you are fully releasing any tension in your pelvic muscles. Failure to do so, even unconsciously, can lead to discomfort or pelvic pain over time.

The mastery of the fundamental Kegel exercises, combined with appropriate breathing and relaxation methods, serves as the initial step towards the restoration of one's pelvic health. Through consistent practice, patience, and conscious control, one shall soon witness the advantages in both their daily activities and overall well-being.

Warming Up

1. Lie down in supine position (on your back) with knees bent and feet on the floor. Perform deep **abdominal breathing** 2-3 times. How to do it? Place both of your hands on your abdomen, just above your belly button. Take a slow deep breath in through your nose; you should feel your abdomen rise as your lungs fill with air; as you slowly exhale through your mouth, allow your abdominal muscles relax; your belly goes back to its normal position. It is important to let your belly to move parallel with the breath and hold the movement until a convenient time. Abdominal breathing helps to relax tense sphincter muscles.

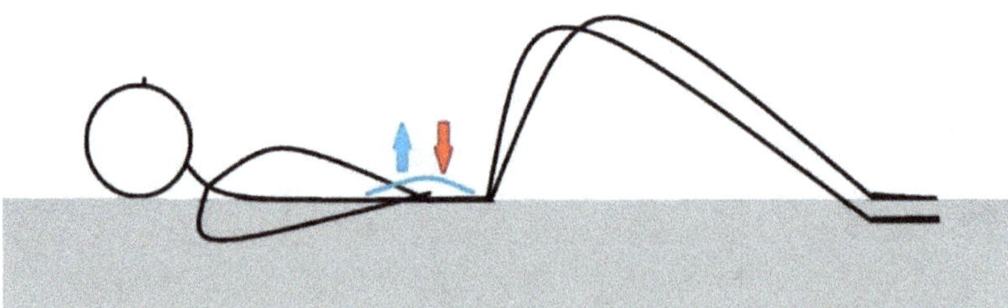

2. Remain in supine position with one leg straight and the other bent at the knee. Shoulders are relaxed, arms by the sides of the body. As you

inhale, gradually raise your extended leg up to hip level by flexing back-and-forth the ankles; then, in a clockwise direction, start to rotate with your raised leg (toes are facing the ceiling) forming small circles, use the hip joint as the axis of rotation. Repeat 5- 5 times the rotation in clockwise and counter-clockwise direction. Try to keep your leg straight. As you exhale slowly, bring your leg back to the mat. Repeat the exercise with your other leg.

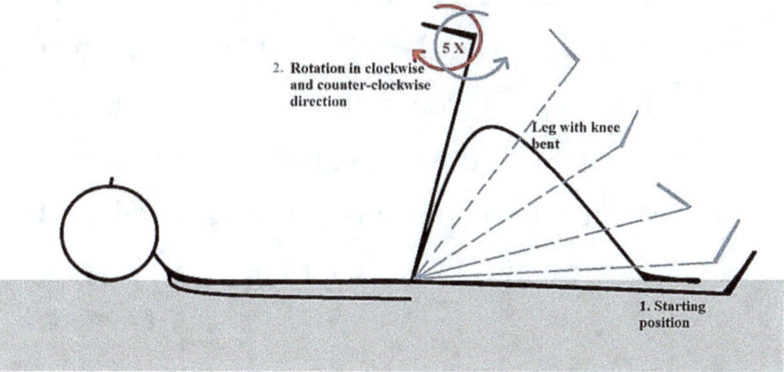

3. In supine position with knees bent, both feet flat on the mat. As you inhale, bring your right knee toward your chest, clasp your hands around the knee and pull it closer to your chest. Hold this position for a few seconds then slowly lower your right leg back to the starting position. Repeat 5 times on each leg, by alternating legs.

At the end, open and close your legs with knees bent, 4-5 times.

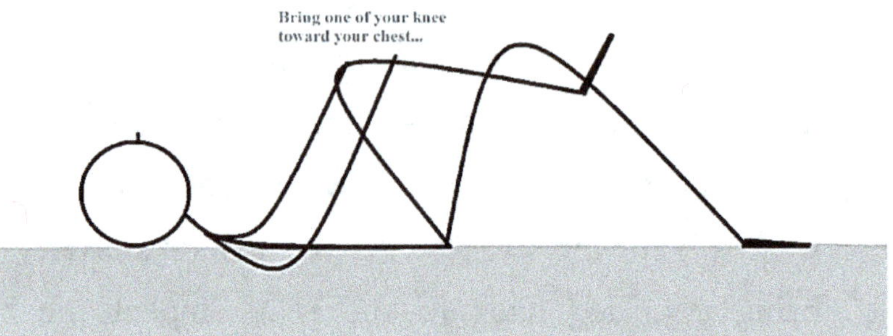

4. In the same position, slowly tighten your buttock muscles, until you feel that these muscles become harder. You can feel the gluteal muscles work if you put your hands in the middle of your buttock. Squeeze your buttocks again, you will feel the muscles go tight and hard under your hands. Relax your muscles.

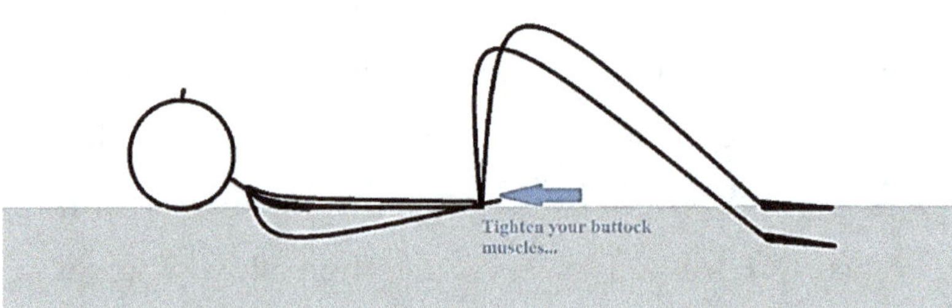

5. Place your hands on your belly, just below your navel and pay attention to your abdominal

muscles. Your abdominal muscles should be soft and relaxed. Muscles should be soft when relaxed. Tightening again your buttock muscles strongly, you should feel that your lower abdominal muscles become a little bit tense as well.

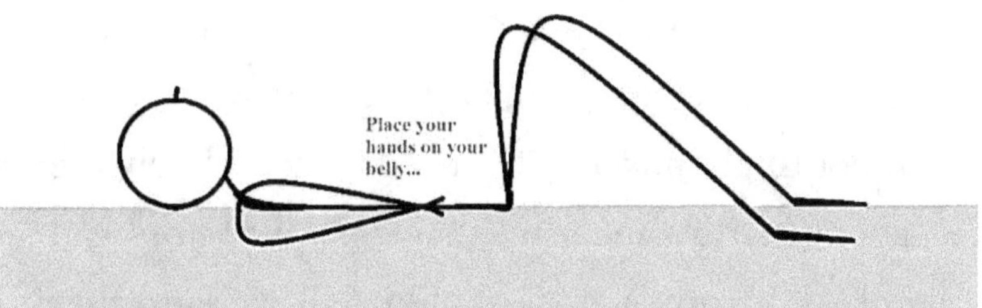

6. Raise your trunk up until your shoulder blades are off the mat. As you lift your trunk off the mat, you should feel a slight burning sensation by the lower abdominal muscles. You should feel as the lower abdominal muscles become a little bit tense. Return to the starting position and relax your muscles.

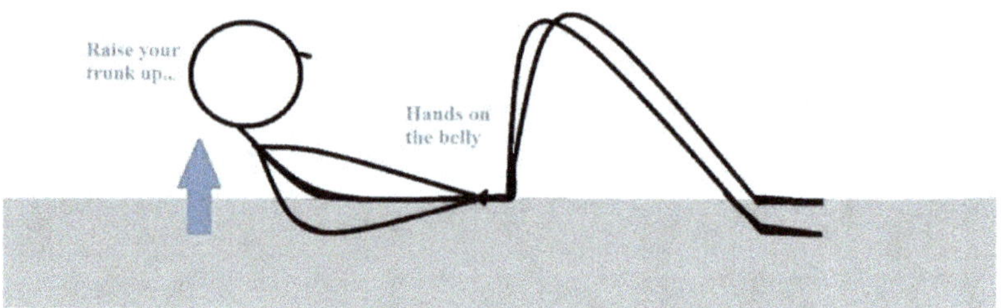

7. Remain in supine position with knees bent; imagine a wet sponge placed between your knees. Place the palms of your hands on your inner thigh muscles. Try to "dry" completely the sponge with squeezing strongly your knees and thighs together. You should feel as the inner thigh muscles become tighter and firmer. When you spread your legs in hip-distance apart, you can feel the inner thigh muscles become relaxed and loose.

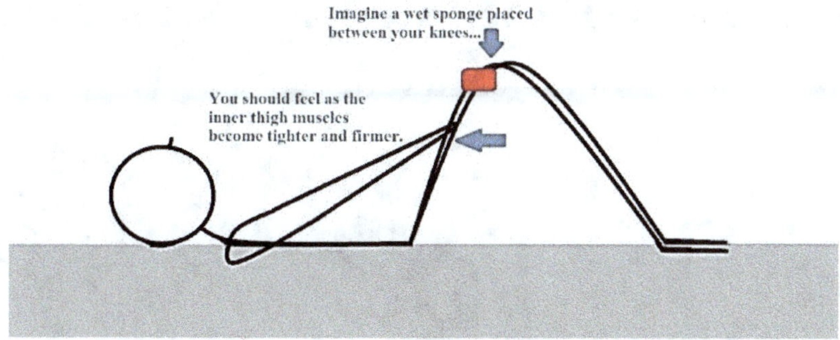

Did you feel with your hand the difference between the tense state and the relaxed state of your muscles?

Exercises To Make Conscious The Movements Of The External Anal Sphincter Muscle

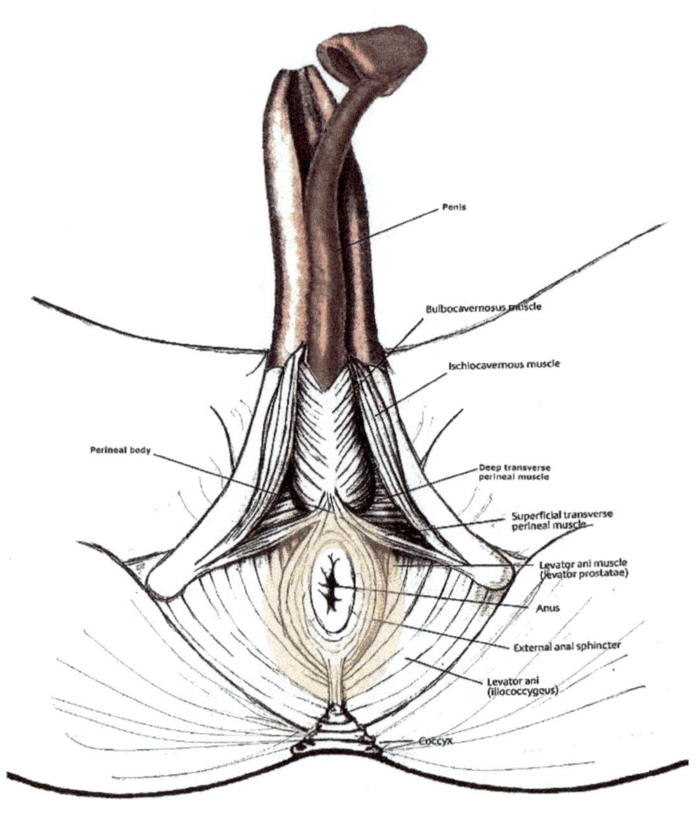

Before commencing pelvic floor exercises, it is crucial to understand and feel the location of the respective muscles. Merely knowing the muscle groups is insufficient; one must have a tangible awareness of their position. The initial attempts to "locate" these muscle systems can be comparable to the challenge of voluntarily wiggling one's ears, as individuals may not have previously considered activating such muscles. However, with appropriate guidance, the identification of the pelvic floor muscles can be a more straightforward process than it may initially appear.

How to Develop Proper Technique for IWT® Pelvic Floor Exercises: Identifying Muscles, Isolation Movement and Breathing

The proper technique for Intimate Wellness Training® (IWT®) pelvic floor exercises entail a methodical and patient approach. The primary objective is to develop a conscious awareness of how to voluntarily contract and relax the sphincter muscle surrounding the anus, the muscles around the penis, and those underlying the prostate. At the outset, the focus should be on isolating each of these muscle groups as much as possible, before progressing to the engagement of the entire pelvic floor musculature as a cohesive unit. Over time, the exercises will become more refined, aimed at building both strength and control within the pelvic floor region. The structure of the IWT® technique can be readily acquired through appropriate instruction. Exercises that may initially appear challenging can be efficiently and securely mastered by all individuals with proper guidance.

Lie on your side with your body in a straight line, keep your bottom leg straight, the upper knee is comfortably flexed and raised toward your chest. Allow your flexed leg to slide in front of the supporting straight leg.

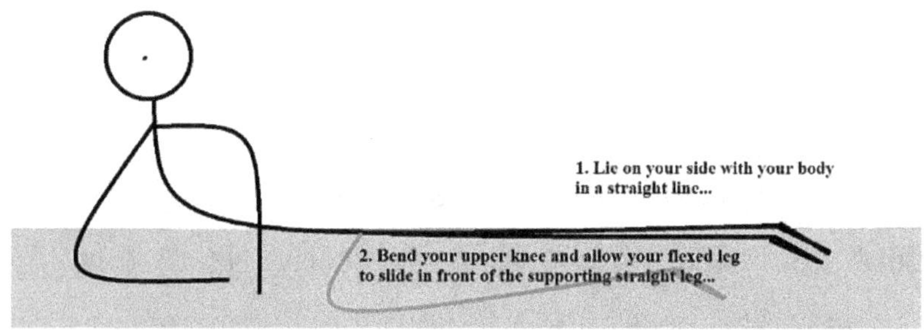

Step 1: Focus on the Anal Sphincter The first area to focus on is the anal orifice. Learning how to properly contract the muscles around the anus is a fundamental step. Start by paying attention to the sensations you feel during anal sphincter contractions, experimenting with different postures until you find the one that allows you to best perceive the movement of the external anal sphincter.

Using Palpation to Build Muscle Awareness Palpation—feeling the muscle contraction with your fingers—is a powerful tool for understanding how your muscles work.

When you feel a muscle contract under your fingertips, it becomes easier to consciously activate that muscle and recognize the difference between a strong and weak contraction, or between contraction and relaxation.

*Place your three central fingertips over the anus from any direction, **over your clothes**. (DO NOT INSERT YOUR FINGER INTO YOUR RECTUM!)*

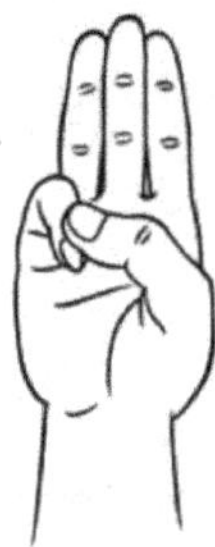

Exercise: Imitating Stool Retention

To begin, perform a movement that mimics the action of retaining stool. Imagine you need to hold back an urgent bowel movement or stop yourself from passing gas. Focus on tightening the sphincter muscle around your anus, engaging it as if you are controlling this urge.

At this point, do not concern yourself with any sensations or movements in the penis or scrotum. Direct all of your attention to the contraction of the anal sphincter and the sensation of tightening beneath your fingertips.

Hold this contraction briefly, and then gently release.

Use your fingertips to feel the contraction of the anal sphincter muscle. This is important for verifying that you are performing the movement correctly, as all other pelvic floor exercises will build upon this basic motion. Perform this imitation of stool retention several times, making sure to "work" only with the perineal muscles, while keeping the surrounding muscles—like the inner thighs, abdomen, and buttocks—relaxed. Only your intimate muscles should be working under your fingertips. Also, remember to breathe normally while squeezing—do not hold your breath.

Don't Be Discouraged

If you can't clearly feel the movement at first, don't be discouraged. Even those with very weak pelvic muscles can learn these exercises. While your pelvic muscles may not be strong enough yet, they will develop with time and practice.

Correct Movements: Signs You're Doing it Right

- **Contraction and Lifting of the Anal Sphincter:** In a correct movement, as you contract the anal sphincter, the anal opening will close tightly, and the circular sphincter muscle will retract upwards toward the abdominal cavity. You can feel this upward, inward movement with your fingertips. Pay attention to how the muscles around your anus tighten as you squeeze and how the anal opening lifts away from your underwear.

- **Inner Buttocks Movement:** If the contraction is correct, the inner parts of your buttocks will slightly move toward each other with each squeeze, though your gluteal muscles should remain as relaxed as possible. While the contraction of the gluteal or inner thigh muscles is not entirely incorrect, it can make learning and isolating the pelvic floor muscles more difficult. To avoid this, start by performing the contraction gently, focusing only on the pelvic muscles.

- **Lower Abdominal Tightening:** During the contraction of the anal sphincter, the lower abdominal muscles (below the belly button) may tighten slightly. This is normal. You may also notice movement in your penis or scrotum, which is fine.

- **Performing the Squeeze Properly:** Focus on performing the retention or closure movement correctly. It's essential to target the right muscles and execute the squeeze accurately to avoid strain or incorrect patterns.

Incorrect Movements: What to Avoid

You are not performing the anal sphincter contraction properly if:

- **Pushing Instead of Lifting:** If you push down on your sphincter muscle instead of squeezing and lifting it up, the anal orifice will open, resembling the action of defecation.

- **Forced Contraction:** Overexerting the circular sphincter muscle can lead to complications like hemorrhoids. Avoid forcing the movement.

- **Chest or Abdominal Tension:** If your chest rises or your upper abdominal muscles (above the belly button) tighten, you are using too much effort. The focus should be on the pelvic muscles, not the upper body.

- **Gluteal Muscle Contraction:** Hardening the gluteal muscles during the exercise is a sign you are not isolating the pelvic muscles properly.

- **Holding Your Breath:** If you find yourself holding your breath while squeezing, remember to breathe naturally throughout the exercise.

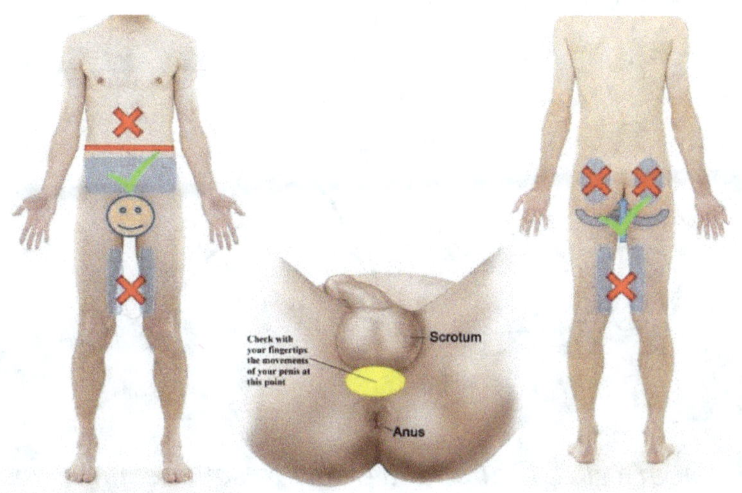

With diligence, equanimity, and meticulous attention, you will command these maneuvers and experience a heightened corporeal awareness. Cultivating appropriate methodology from the outset guarantees the capacity to safely and efficiently develop strength in the pelvic musculature, culminating in enhanced bladder regulation, sexual vigor, and core stability.

Check out the squeeze of the anal sphincter also in supine position.

Lie on your back with knees bent, feet flat on the floor. Place knees and feet hip-distance apart, arms beside your body.

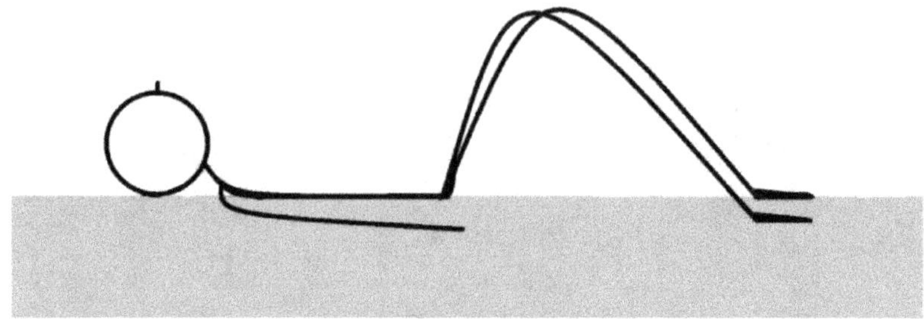

**Repeat the exercise described above also in all fours
position, the thighs and arms upright, keep your back
and shoulders straight.**

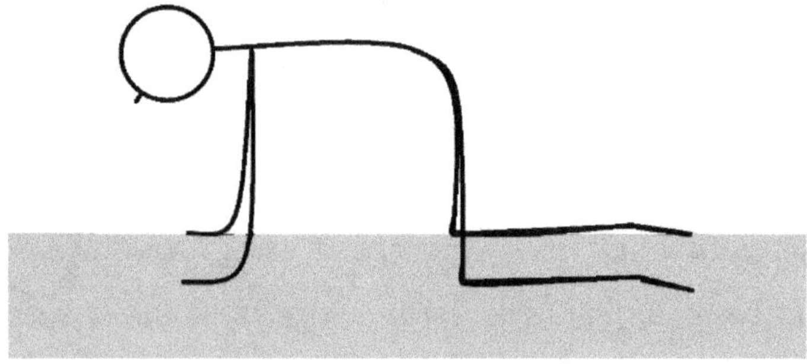

Now settle yourself into that position, in which you have felt better the movements of the anal sphincter muscle or in which you could tighten the muscles around your anus firmly.

You can assume the supine position with knees bent, the side-lying position, or the "on all fours" position.

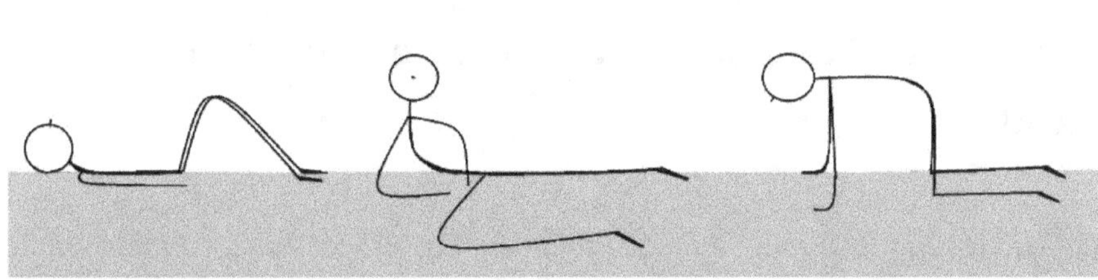

The comfortable posture is important, because if you feel uncomfortable in a posture while doing these exercises, then you are unable to focus on what you are doing.

If you cannot decide, I suggest you to settle yourself in supine position with knees bent. In the supine position, the muscles of the pelvic floor are less stressed.

Mastering the Maximum Squeeze and Relaxation Technique

In this step, you will focus on squeezing the circular sphincter muscle around the anus, similar to the previous exercise, but this time with maximum force—this is known as the "maximum squeeze."

The capacity of a muscle to contract is contingent upon its length and the extent of the contraction. For the purpose of muscular strength and development, the contraction should be executed with maximum exertion. Only the muscle fibers that are fully engaged during the exercise will become strengthened, which is why it is imperative to contract the anal sphincter muscle as forcefully as possible. While undertaking this contraction, it is advisable to maintain steady and relaxed breathing, refraining from holding one's breath.

Important!
Make sure that your contraction is focused on the hidden pelvic floor muscles, specifically those located between your legs. Avoid tightening your buttocks, inner thighs, or pulling in your abdomen. In the beginning, it may be helpful to use your hands for guidance. Place your hands on your buttocks or inner thighs to ensure that you are activating only your pelvic floor muscles.

If your facial expression alters during the contraction of the pelvic muscles, such as when exerting effort due to constipation, you are applying an excessive amount of force during the maximum contraction. When instructed to "contract your pelvic floor muscles as much as possible," I intend for only the intimate muscles to be engaged. Your facial expression should remain unchanged throughout the maximum contraction.

Exercise: Focusing on the Anal Sphincter Muscle
Begin by relaxing your abdominal muscles completely. Direct your attention solely to the ring of muscles surrounding your anus, known as the **anal sphincter**. Gently contract this muscle by **squeezing it tightly**, as though you are trying to pull it upward and inward. Visualize lifting the muscle up deeper into your body.

Once you have engaged the muscle, see if you can increase the strength of the contraction slightly more, pulling the sphincter muscle even further inward. **Hold this contraction briefly**.

Now, **slowly release the tension**, allowing the muscle to relax fully. As you relax, take a long, slow exhale—almost like a soft sigh of relief. You should feel a noticeable sense of letting go, both in your muscle and your breath.

If you have chosen another position before, for the next exercise, please settle yourself in supine position with knees bent.

Exercise: Focusing on Relaxation After Contraction
Now, repeat the previous exercise, engaging in a strong contraction of your anal sphincter muscle. This time,

however, focus not just on the contraction but also on how the pelvic muscles return to their relaxed state afterward.

As you release the contraction, pay close attention to the sensation of the muscle gradually letting go. You should feel the tension easing as your anal sphincter returns to its natural, relaxed state—moving gently downward, as if toward your underwear. During this relaxation phase, you should have a clear, noticeable feeling of letting go.

Take your time to fully experience this process.

No Need to Worry About "Accidents"

Relaxing your anal sphincter muscle during these exercises will not cause any "accidents." In fact, for evacuation (like bowel movements) to occur, both the external and internal anal sphincters must relax, and the internal sphincter operates involuntarily, responding only to the evacuation reflex.

The Importance of Relaxation

In pelvic floor exercises, relaxation is just as important as contraction. During contraction, the increased pressure restricts blood flow, reducing the supply of oxygen and nutrients to the muscles. However, when you fully relax the muscles, blood circulation improves, delivering vital nutrients and oxygen, which supports muscle recovery and prepares them for the next contraction. If you contract your pelvic floor muscles without fully relaxing them, they may remain slightly tense, limiting blood flow and hindering muscle development.

It's not uncommon for the relaxation phase to be more challenging than the contraction itself. If your muscles still feel tense after contraction, it may feel like an unpleasant sensation of tightness. To assist in relaxation, try gently separating your knees as wide as comfortable or practicing abdominal breathing (refer to the warm-up section for more details).

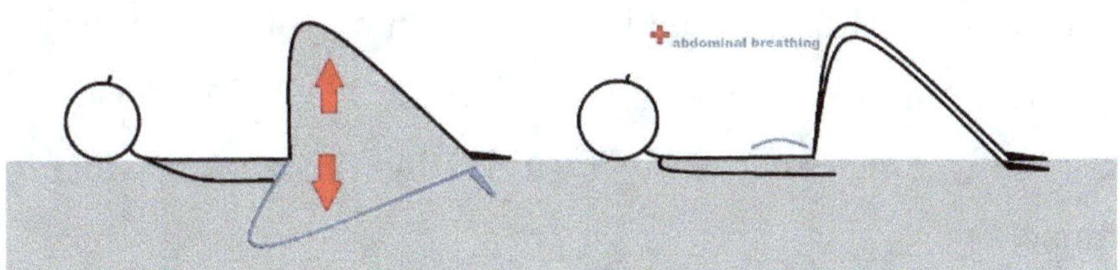

Elevator Kegel - Steps for a Maximum Anal Sphincter Squeeze and Relaxation

Until now, you had to pay attention how your external anal sphincter muscle can be tightened and relaxed. Now you should perform the contraction of the anal sphincter muscle slowly, gradually and consciously, observing the phases of the contraction. The contraction of the anal sphincter muscle should be gradual from the relaxed state of the muscle until reaching the maximal strength of contraction without stopping at the different phases of the contraction!

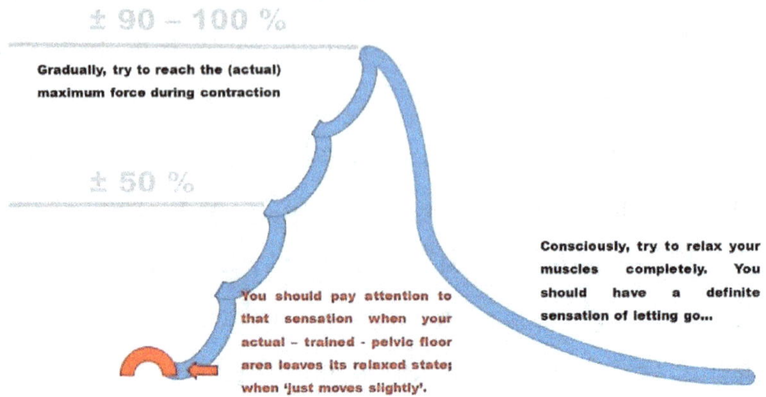

Imagine your pelvic floor muscles are an elevator. Slowly lift them to the "first floor" (gentle contraction), then the "second floor" (stronger contraction), and finally to the "third floor" (full contraction). As soon as you arrive to the "third floor", start lower the elevator back down slowly gradually and consciously by relaxing the anal sphincter muscle.

1. **Start with Relaxation:** Ensure the anal sphincter muscle is in a completely relaxed state.

2. **Engage Slightly:** Begin to contract the muscle gently, paying close attention to the feeling when the sphincter muscle just starts to engage.

3. **Increase Force Gradually:** Continue squeezing the sphincter until you reach about half of your maximum strength.

4. **Approach Maximum Force:** Continue to tighten the muscle until you feel you are contracting with almost maximum force.

5. **Reach Maximum Contraction:** Squeeze as tightly as you can, reaching your maximum contraction.

6. **Relax Fully:** Once you have held the maximum squeeze, release the contraction and allow the muscles to relax completely.

Don't Worry if You Lose Strength

If the strength of your contraction fades during the exercise, don't worry—just squeeze your sphincter again and continue. It's perfectly normal, especially if your pelvic floor muscles are not yet strong enough to maintain the contraction. At first, it may be challenging to perform this exercise successfully due to weak pelvic floor muscles. However, managing a gradual contraction usually will be easier as your pelvic muscles become stronger. When your pelvic muscles become stronger, you will find it easier to maintain the contraction for longer periods. Finally, the ability to relax your muscles gradually and slowly will develop over time, typically as one of the last skills.

Exercise: Endurance Hold Kegel

Repeat the previous exercise, but this time focus on building endurance in your pelvic floor muscles.

- Begin by **slowly contracting** the anal sphincter, gradually increasing the intensity of the contraction **over a count of four**.
- Once you reach the maximum level of contraction, **hold the tension for another count of four**, maintaining the strongest squeeze you can manage.
- After holding, begin to **gradually release** the contraction, allowing your muscles to relax slowly **over a count of four**.

Focus on controlling both the contraction and the release, aiming for smooth and even movements throughout the exercise. Remember, the goal here is not only to strengthen your pelvic floor but also to improve your muscle endurance and control.

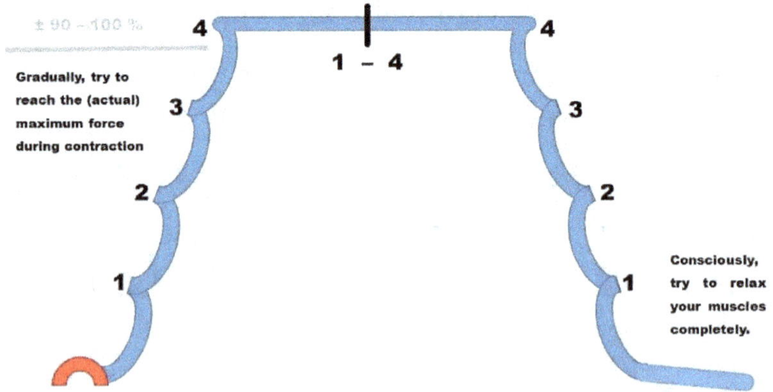

Next Step: Combining Contraction with a Posterior Pelvic Tilt

Once you have mastered the maximum squeeze, the next step is to perform the anal sphincter contraction while engaging in a posterior pelvic tilt, which adds a new layer of challenge and effectiveness to your pelvic floor training.

How to Perform a Posterior Pelvic Tilt

A posterior pelvic tilt involves flattening the curve of your lower back.

Posterior Pelvic Tilt

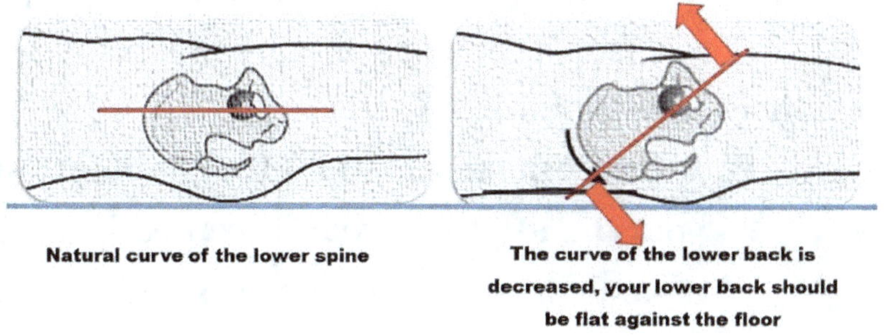

Let's walk through the movement of the pelvis step by step. Pay careful attention to the sequence of the movement:

In a Supine Position

1. **Start with Breathing:**
   - Lie on your back with your knees bent and feet flat on the floor.
   - First, take a deep breath in. As you exhale, begin the pelvic tilt movement.

2. **Pelvic Tilt Movement:**
   - As you exhale, **slowly tilt your pelvis backwards**. The goal is to flatten your lower back against the mat by <u>tightening your abdominal muscles</u> and tilting your pelvis slightly upward.
   - Your buttocks should remain on the floor—do not lift them.
   - While you exhale, your abdomen should naturally move towards your spine, helping you flatten the curve in your lower back.

3. **Check the Position:**
   - In this position, **you should not be able to slip your hand** under your lower back, as the natural curve of your lumbar spine will have straightened. **Check it!** If your lower back is pressed into the mat correctly, your hand won't fit beneath it.

4. **Return to Neutral:**

o   At the end of the exhalation, relax and allow your spine and pelvis to return to their original, neutral position.

! Do not hold your breath while performing the pelvic tilt.

Practice Makes Perfect

Repeat the pelvic tilt movement a few times until you feel confident with it. Although the movement might seem simple, it can be surprisingly challenging to master, especially when done correctly. Be patient with yourself, it gets easier with practice!

Posterior Pelvic Tilt Plus: Adding More Intensity

Once you have gotten comfortable with the basic posterior pelvic tilt, it's time to intensify the contraction by integrating the **"Posterior Pelvic Tilt Plus"**. This version engages both your pelvic floor muscles and your gluteal muscles for a deeper contraction.

In a Supine Position with Knees Bent, Feet on the Floor:

1. **Engage Your Gluteal Muscles:**
   o   Begin by **squeezing your gluteal (buttock) muscles** together slightly.

2. **Start the Pelvic Tilt:**
   o   As you squeeze your glutes, **tilt your pelvis backward** and press your lower back firmly

against the mat, flattening the curve in your lumbar spine.

3. **Check the Position:**
    - o Just like before, in this position, **you should not be able to slip your hand under your lower back. Check again!** The lower back should remain flat on the mat.

4. **Deepen the Contraction:**
    - o Gradually **increase the squeeze of your glutes** to maximum force. As you do this, you will feel your belly retract toward your spine, and the contraction will feel stronger and deeper.

5. **Exhale and Relax:**
    - o As you exhale, slowly relax your glutes and pelvic floor muscles, allowing your spine and pelvis to return to their neutral position.

POSTERIOR PELVIC TILT +

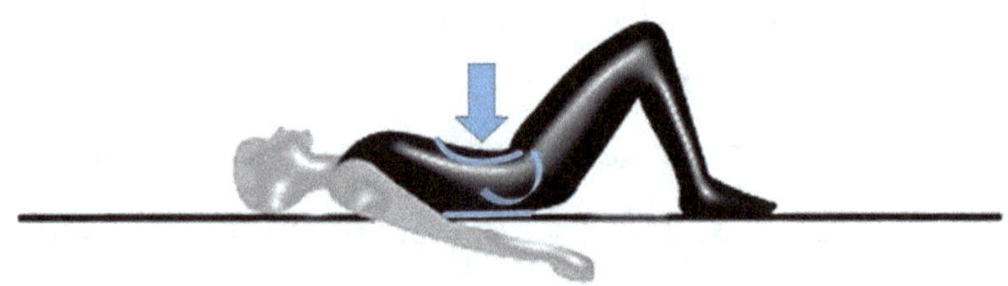

Practice and Breathe

Repeat this movement several times, focusing on both the contraction and relaxation phases. Don't forget to keep your breathing steady throughout the exercise!

Combining the Posterior Pelvic Tilt Plus with Anal Sphincter Contraction

Now, we will take it a step further by integrating the contraction of the anal sphincter muscle with the contraction of your buttock muscles. This combination intensifies the workout, giving your pelvic floor muscles more strength and control.

Earlier, I instructed you to avoid using your gluteal muscles so that you could first learn to isolate and move your **anal sphincter** muscle voluntarily. Now that you have practiced that, we can combine these movements for a more powerful contraction.

Let's join the pelvic tilt + with the contraction of the anal sphincter muscle in practice!

Exercise: Full Pelvic Engagement with Relaxation

- Begin by **relaxing your abdominal** muscles completely. Focus solely on the movement of your anal sphincter muscle.

- Gently tighten the **muscles around your anus**, creating a slight tension. Hold this tension while **squeezing your buttock** muscles together slightly. As you do this, **tilt your pelvis backward**, pressing your lower back down into the mat beneath you.

- Gradually **increase the contraction** of your buttock muscles, building up to your maximum strength. Simultaneously, squeeze your anal sphincter as strongly as possible, pulling the muscles up and inward. Check to see if you can intensify the contraction even further.

- As you exhale, **release all the tension**. Allow your anal and buttock muscles to soften and relax your abdominal muscles fully. Take a slow, elongated exhale, almost like a sigh of relief.

- Let your spine and pelvis naturally return to their original, neutral position.

Repeat the previous task with a pelvic tilt + but try to keep the maximal contraction for a count of 4.

Next exercise to close the section:

Pelvic Floor Activation and Bridge Exercise

Position: Remain in a **supine position** (lying on your back), with your **knees bent** and feet flat on the floor. To help maintain balance, place your **arms alongside your body**, palms facing down.

- Begin by performing **8 quick, strong squeezes** with your **anal sphincter muscle, as quickly as you can**. These should be fast, definite contractions—**squeeze and release** without holding the contraction. Stay relaxed and focused on the movement.

Bridge Pose: As you **exhale**, press your feet onto the floor and **slowly lift your pelvis** off the mat. Raise your hips until your body forms a straight line from your **shoulders to your knees**, maintaining your pelvis in a neutral position. Hold this bridge for **5-10 seconds**, ensuring you continue to **breathe deeply and steadily** throughout.

Release: After the hold, **slowly roll your spine back down** to the floor, vertebra by vertebra. Once fully lowered, take a deep breath in through your nose, allowing your abdomen to rise. As you **exhale slowly**, relax your pelvic muscles completely. This deep, abdominal breathing helps release any tension in muscles not under your direct control, promoting full relaxation.

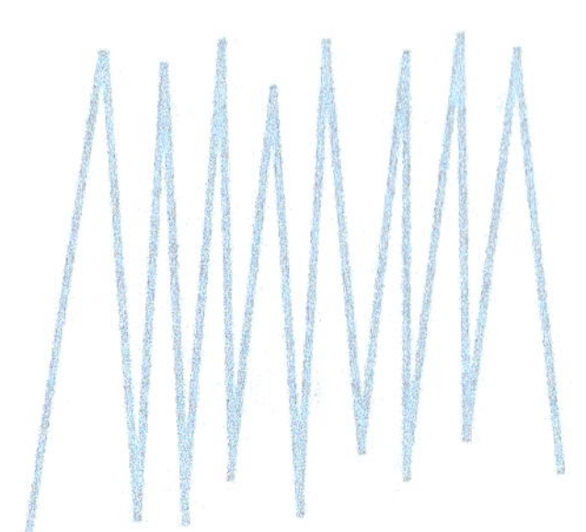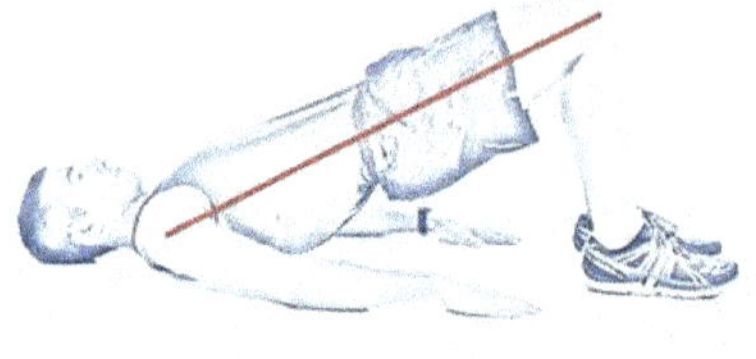

If you cannot hold this position, as an alternative you can place a cushion under your buttocks for a few seconds to keep them raised

Keep in Mind!

Even when performing a maximum squeeze, the work should come primarily from your pelvic floor muscles, not from other surrounding muscles. Your goal is to focus on isolating and strengthening this critical muscle group while enhancing the intensity of the exercise with your glutes.

By practicing this combination regularly, you will strengthen both your pelvic floor and anal sphincter muscles, helping you achieve greater control, endurance, and overall pelvic health.

Exercises To Make Conscious The Movements Of The Muscles Around The Penis And Under The Prostate Gland

In this section, the focus will be on replicating nearly identical exercises concentrating on the musculature surrounding the penis, the rectum, and the region beneath the prostate gland. While it may appear unconventional to emphasize the training of these specific muscle groups, maintaining the strength and integrity of these muscles is pivotal to their proper physiological function, even as one progresses through the aging process. A robust pelvic floor can contribute to preserving the height and fullness of penile erections throughout an individual's lifetime. Conversely, without consistent exercise, the lateral muscles may weaken, potentially leading to a gradual decline in the angle of erection. Furthermore, suboptimal blood circulation within the penis can negatively impact one's sexual vitality.

Position yourself on knee-elbow position. Keep your legs and knees in hip distance apart, to be able to palpate the muscles at the base of your penis.

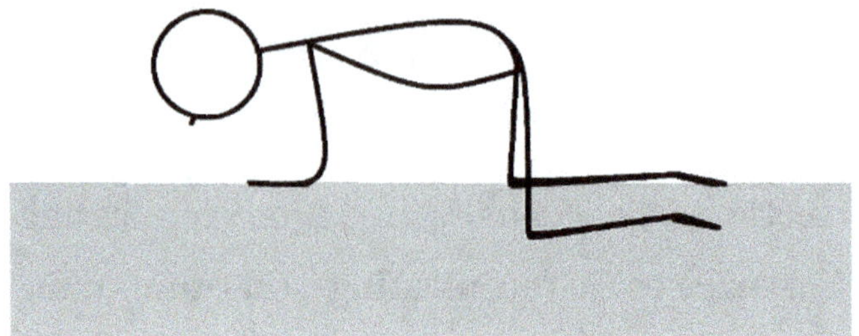

Place your three middle fingertips at the base of your penis, close to the scrotum, over your clothes. Stay in a knee-elbow position.

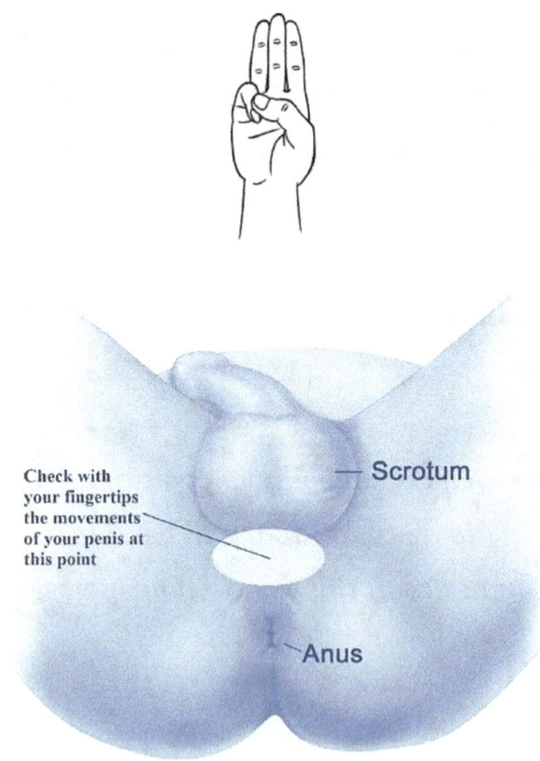

Now, focus on the movements of your penis while rhythmically tightening your anal sphincter muscle. As you do this, pay attention to how the muscles around and within your penis contract and relax in parallel. This exercise helps you build awareness and control over these muscles, which is key to improving both strength and circulation.

Here is the **exercise** to start with:

- **Start with Relaxation**: Relax your abdominal muscles completely.
- Begin by **rhythmically squeezing your anal sphincter muscle**, similar to how you would blink your eyes quickly. Squeeze and relax the muscles around your **anus** repeatedly. While doing this, observe the sensations in your **penis**. Pay attention to what you perceive under your fingertips.
- After a few contractions, **hold the squeeze** of your anal sphincter muscle for a moment.
- As you **relax your anal sphincter**, notice how the muscles around and in your penis become also relaxed. What do you feel around and in your penis when you release the tension in your anus?

Important Note:

Do not tighten your buttocks, inner thigh muscles, or pull in your abdomen!

Next Step

In the same position, you will now imitate the muscle movement used to stop urine flow. This might be a bit tricky, as you may notice your anal sphincter muscle moving as well. However, focus entirely on the muscles around your urethra in your penis, ignoring the anal sphincter's movement.

1. **Relax your abdominal muscles.** To engage the muscles at the base of your penis, simulate the contraction you would use to consciously stop urine flow. Imagine someone walking into the bathroom while you are urinating, and you need to immediately stop the flow, and then start it again. Squeeze the muscles <u>rhythmically</u>—the ones you would use to hold back urine. If you are doing it correctly, you should feel the base of your penis move slightly upward, toward your abdomen each time you tighten your pelvic floor muscles.

2. **Pay attention to the movements under your fingertips.** After a few contractions, **hold the squeeze** for a moment.

3. As you **relax the muscles**, focus on how the muscles around and within your penis let go. You should feel

a pleasant sensation of relaxation. This release, or "letting go," is an important part of the exercise.

Note: You can test this movement by stopping your urine flow "for real", to identify the correct muscles. However, do this test only once to avoid retaining urine or disrupting normal bladder emptying. Once you are sure you have found the right muscles, ensure your bladder is completely emptied and relaxed.

Correct Movements:

- **Focus on the muscles around your penis.** When you contract these muscles, it should feel similar to the sensation of squeezing the base of the penis with your hand.
- **Synchronized contraction.** As you contract your anal sphincter, the muscles around your penis will also engage. You will notice that as your anus tightens and relaxes rhythmically, the muscles around and within your penis follow the same pattern. The warmth generated by the activity of the pelvic floor muscles can help you recognize the correct muscles.
- **Physical sensations.** You might feel your penis "pull in" slightly, and your scrotum will lift up a bit. With each contraction, your penis may twitch or draw inward toward your body, while the muscles at the

base tighten and move slightly backward, toward your rectum.

- **Visual feedback.** If you stand naked in front of a mirror and contract the right muscles, you should see the base of your penis draw in, and your scrotum lift up slightly.

Incorrect Movements:

- **Anal orifice movement.** If you feel your anal opening widen, as though preparing for evacuation, or if it moves downward, that is an incorrect movement.
- **Belly tension.** Avoid pulling your belly inward during the exercise. Doing so can mistakenly tense up the muscles around your penis, which disrupts the correct muscle engagement.

Now, please lie on your back with knees bent. Make sure you feel comfortable.

Coordinating Pelvic Floor Muscle Areas

You have now observed the movements of the anal sphincter and the muscles around the penis separately. In this exercise, you will focus on how these two muscle groups work together. Think of the area as resembling the number 8-two overlapping circles. The point where these two areas connect is just below the prostate gland. This is the deepest part of the pelvic floor, linking the muscles around the penis, anus, and the muscles beneath the prostate.

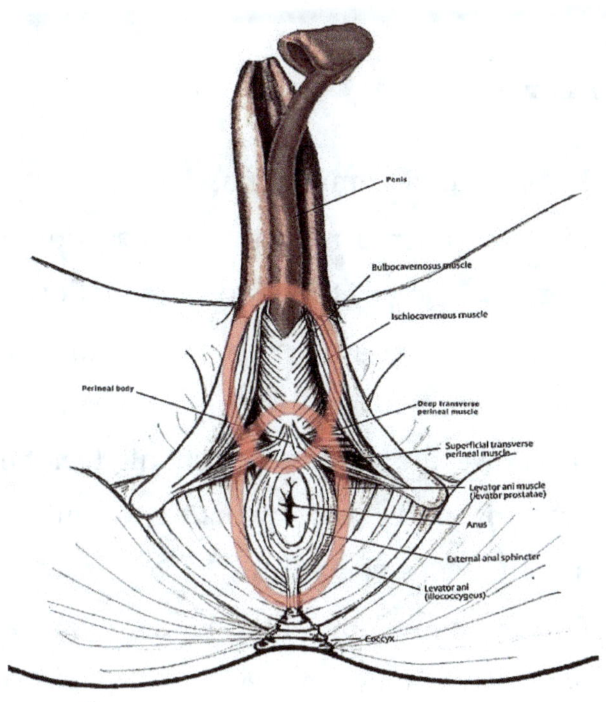

The pelvic floor functions as a unified, elastic band of muscles—like a hammock. When one side of the muscle group moves, the other side reacts. If you contract the muscles around the penis (the front circle) and the anus (the rear circle), the center point between them, near the prostate, will also rise.

You can contract both areas simultaneously or focus on one and then the other. Both methods are effective. The goal is to **pay attention** to both areas as they contract and relax.

Exercise Instructions:

- Relax your abdominal muscles.
- First, perform a moderate contraction, as if you were consciously trying to stop the flow of urine,
- while in parallel start also mimicking the movement you use to stop passing gas or holding in a bowel movement. You should feel the muscles around both the penis and anus tighten simultaneously.
- Once you are sure both areas are engaged, relax your pelvic floor muscles.

Repeat the exercise, but this time **focus** on the point below the prostate gland. Notice how it lifts as you contract and returns to its normal position when you relax.

Now, **repeat the exercise** again, but this time try tightening the muscles around your penis **with maximum effort**. Engage every muscle that contributes to the contraction, pushing yourself to your limit (only with your pelvic floor muscles!!!). Pay attention to how much you can contract the muscles around your penis.

Maximizing Muscle Contractions for Pelvic Floor Strength

As I mentioned earlier, a muscle fiber only strengthens when it is fully contracted. Partial or weak contractions leave the weakest parts of the muscle underworked, preventing them from gaining strength. This is why it is important to engage the full range of the pelvic floor muscles during each exercise.

Refining the Contraction:

As you contract the muscles, observe each movement carefully. Check if you can tighten the muscles even further by lifting your scrotum slightly more or pulling the base of your penis a bit closer to your rectum.

These are subtle movements. Your penis will not shift dramatically, but these small adjustments help improve the effectiveness of your pelvic floor muscle contractions. Think of them as checkpoints to enhance the quality of your exercise.

Exercise Instructions:
Focus on the muscles around the penis.

- **Relax** your abdominal muscles.
- Begin by gently **squeezing the muscles around your penis**, as if trying to stop the flow of urine. Use moderate force—don't strain. **Pay attention** to how the muscles contract around the penis. You might feel a tightening sensation, almost as if the muscles are closing in a circular shape. You may also notice the base of the penis feels like it's being squeezed, similar to pressing toothpaste from a tube.
- If you feel this contraction, particularly at the base of the penis or if your scrotum lifts, **hold the contraction briefly**.
- Then, like pulling back a car's old-school gearstick, **tighten further** by pulling the base of your penis back toward the rectum and lifting the scrotum even more.
- Now, **relax**. Let your abdominal muscles go soft and release the pelvic floor muscles. Take a slow, deep exhale, like a sigh of relief, and feel your muscles let go completely.

Note: Avoid holding your breath, tightening your buttocks, squeezing your legs together, or pulling in your abdomen. Focus only on using your internal pelvic muscles.

Pay attention to relaxation.

Repeat the exercise, but this time, consciously **focus on the relaxation** of the muscles. Feel how the tension around and inside the penis, as well as under the prostate, fades away. Notice how the scrotum descends back to its normal position.

To ensure the urethra relaxes, let your belly soften completely. You may have already noticed that when you contract your pelvic floor muscles, your lower abdominal muscles also tense up slightly. These muscles work together with the pelvic floor, even when relaxing. The sensation of urethral relaxation is similar to the pleasant feeling that comes after urination.

Note: Do not use your buttock or inner thigh muscles during this exercise. It is also important not to pull in your abdomen, as this will cause the muscles around the penis to tense up involuntarily.

Next step. Perform a gradual contraction and release.

Now, squeeze the muscles around your penis **with awareness.** Slowly and gradually build up the **contraction** to your maximum force, **counting to 4. Hold** this strongest squeeze **for a count of 4.** Then, slowly and gradually **relax** the muscles, **counting to 4** again. As you relax, exhale slowly and deeply, almost like a sigh. This prolonged exhalation helps activate the parasympathetic nervous system, which promotes relaxation throughout the body, including the pelvic muscles.

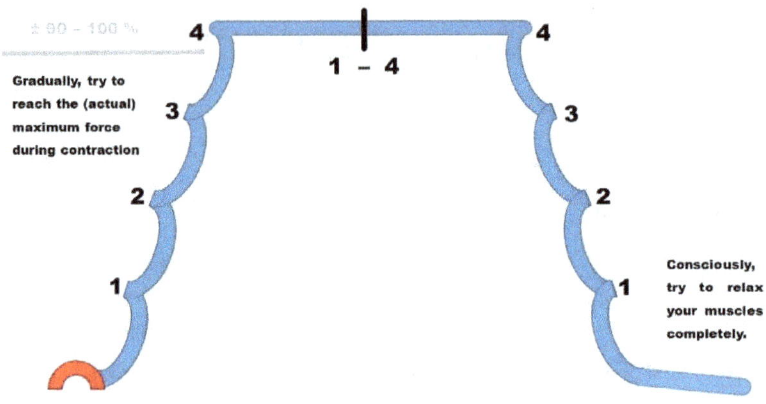

Note: Always make sure your abdominal muscles are relaxed before tightening the pelvic floor muscles.

Anterior Pelvic Tilt Exercise:

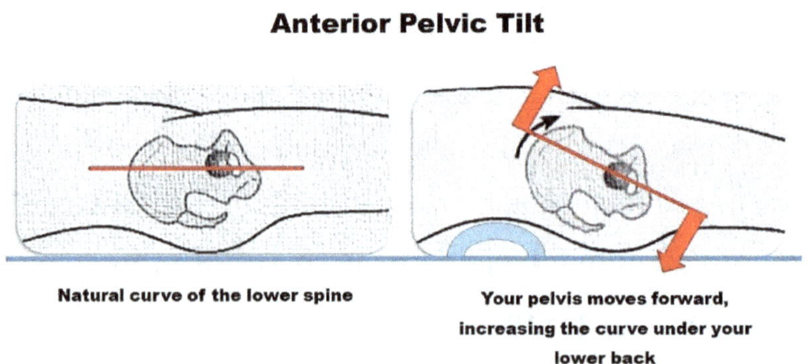

How do I do an anterior pelvic tilt? An anterior pelvic tilt is the opposite movement of posterior pelvic tilt, which means that your pelvis moves forward, increasing the curve under your lower back. By incorporating these pelvic tilts into your routine, you will improve not only your pelvic floor strength but also your overall core stability. In standing position, if the abdomen protrudes forward contributing to an imbalance in the muscles in the pelvis and hip area. Excessive anterior pelvic tilt can contribute greatly to postural dysfunction like lower back pain, knee pain, flat feet, hip pain etc. In this exercise, the anterior pelvic tilt in supine position will be applied for therapeutic purpose.

Let's see the **exercise** with the movement of the pelvis. Pay careful attention to the sequence of the movements:

Lie on your back with your knees bent and feet flat on the floor.

- Relax your abdominal muscles.
- Slightly squeeze the muscles around and in your penis and hold this tension.
- Tilt your pelvis forward, creating a small "bridge" under your lower back (you should be able to insert your hand under your spine).
- Increase the force of the contraction of the muscles around your penis to maximum force, squeeze your

penis tightly, "lift" the scrotum up as high as you can, "pull back" the base of your penis toward the rectum.

- Hold for a count of 4, then slowly relax the muscles while exhaling. Let your pelvis and spine return to their neutral position.

ANTERIOR PELVIC TILT

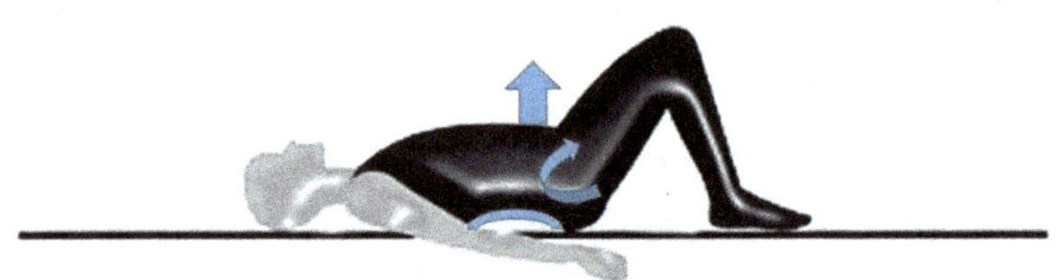

Perform the pelvic tilt a few times or until you feel confident with the movement.

! Do not hold your breath while performing the pelvic tilt.

Strengthening the deepest part of the Perineum

The next exercise is highly beneficial for supporting prostate and testicular health. By creating alternating movements in front of and behind the prostate, you can gently massage the prostate internally. This helps to improve blood circulation, relieve the symptoms of prostatitis, and ease muscular tension.

Understanding the Prostate's Position and Why It is Vulnerable

The prostate gland is situated in a suboptimal anatomical position. It is located between two "storage areas"- the urinary bladder and the rectum, subjected to consistent pressure from above by the weight of the bladder and from below by the pelvic floor muscles. Additionally, the prostate bears pressure from prolonged sitting, particularly in the case of poor posture, which increases intra-abdominal pressure. Furthermore, the urethra traverses directly through the prostate. Prolonged sitting or improper posture can lead to stagnant blood flow to the prostate, enabling bacteria to settle and causing inflammation (prostatitis).

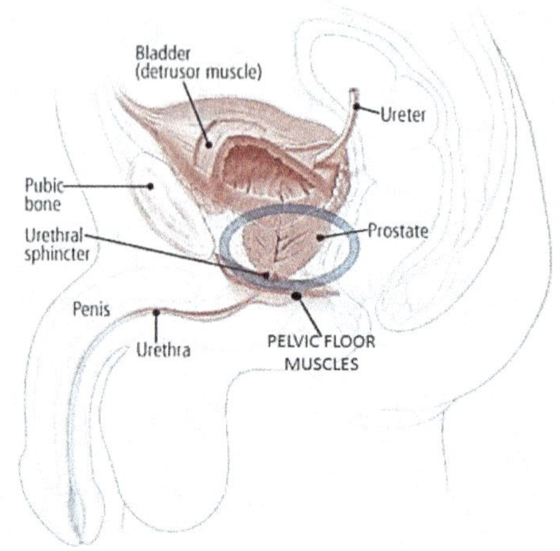

Due to this compromised circulation, antibiotics often struggle to effectively penetrate the prostate. Dehydration may also contribute to prostatitis by producing concentrated urine, which can irritate the prostate and urinary tract, leading to inflammation or discomfort. Insufficient hydration also reduces the body's ability to flush out bacteria and toxins, increasing the risk of infection in the prostate gland. Maintaining adequate hydration supports prostate health by promoting better urinary flow and reducing the likelihood of urinary and prostate complications. Erectile dysfunction is a common issue among men with sedentary occupations, and these problems are frequently accompanied by chronic prostatitis. Stress worsens the situation since it may intensify the tension of the pelvic floor musculature, thereby diminishing the circulatory flow.

The Role of Pelvic Floor Exercises in Prostate Health

Pelvic floor exercises constitute one of the most effective means of addressing prostate inflammation. By enhancing blood circulation in the pelvic area, these exercises prevent the accumulation of pathogens and facilitate the relaxation of tense pelvic muscles. All prostate disorders stemming from impaired circulation can be alleviated through these exercises specifically tailored for men. The more forceful the contraction of the pelvic floor muscles, the more pronounced the beneficial effect. However, if one is afflicted with prostatitis, this exercise may initially induce discomfort or even pain. While mild discomfort is natural and typically subsides over time, during an acute episode of prostatitis, it is advisable to perform these exercises at a moderate intensity to minimize excessive discomfort.

Balance scale exercise Step-by-Step Instructions:

Starting Position:
Lie in a supine position with your knees bent. In earlier exercises, you may have noticed how the anal sphincter muscle and the muscles around the base of the penis work with varying intensity. In this exercise, you will **alternately engage the muscles** around your penis (the anterior muscles), and the anal sphincter muscle (the posterior

muscles). Begin with a small or moderate squeeze of the muscles around your penis, followed by a squeeze of the anal sphincter, one after the other. The goal is to lift the anterior part of the pelvic floor (the muscles around your penis) first, then the posterior part (anal muscles). Alternate between these two contractions, repeating the movement a few times.

Focus on Sensations:

As you alternate the contractions between the muscles around your penis and anal contractions, notice the gentle rocking sensation in your perineum. You may feel that the muscles under the prostate don't tighten with equal strength. This is normal. With practice, you can gradually increase the intensity of these contractions, but in the beginning, focus on small, controlled movements. Focus on the sensation of alternating between stronger contractions of the muscles around your penis and the muscles around the anus, as if your perineum is gently rocking back and forth.

Squeeze the muscles around the penis:

Now, perform a small **squeeze around the penis, holding the contraction for a count of 4**. Pay attention to the anterior part of the prostate during this time. As you **relax** the muscles, notice where you feel a pleasant sensation—this awareness helps you connect with the movement.

Anal Squeeze:

Next, focus on the muscles around the anus. Slightly **squeeze the anal opening, holding the tension for a count of 4,** then **relax** the anal sphincter while paying attention to the posterior part of the prostate. As you relax the anal muscles, once again, pay attention where you feel any pleasant sensations during this relaxation phase.

Balanced Movements:

You may observe that the part of perineum under the prostate does not tense up with equal force during this exercise. The important thing is to focus on the alternating sensations, sometimes the anterior part of the prostate contracts more intensely, other times the anal sphincter does (the posterior part). It should feel like your perineum is gently swinging or rocking back and forth.

Direction of Movement:

When you focus on the squeeze around the penis, you may notice that the penis seems to move upwards, towards the abdominal cavity. On the other hand, when the movement is led by the anal sphincter, the penis moves downward. The balance point between these movements is in the central point of the perineum, just under the prostate.

Rhythm and Control:

Some men prefer to perform this exercise with fast contractions, while others find slow, deliberate contractions more beneficial. During the learning phase, rhythm is less important than focusing on how the muscles tense up during contractions. Although all the perineal muscles are working together, the emphasis should be on the direction of movement and the varying intensity of the PC (pubococcygeus) muscle contractions.

Building Strength Over Time:

This exercise will evolve into a strengthening routine once you are able to perform it with maximum force. However, it is crucial not to attempt maximum force until you have built sufficient muscle control through moderate or small contractions. Starting with too much intensity too soon could lead to muscle strain. During the learning phase, stick to gentle or moderate contractions, and only increase the intensity once you are confident in your technique and muscle awareness. Be sure to maintain awareness of your breathing and avoid tensing your abdominal muscles or legs during these exercises. Remember, consistent practice will help you strengthen your pelvic floor muscles, leading to better bladder control, improved sexual function, and overall core stability.

Next **exercise** to close the section:

Pelvic Floor Activation and Bridge Exercise

Position: Remain in a **supine position** (lying on your back), with your knees bent and feet flat on the floor. To help maintain balance, place your arms alongside your body, palms facing down.

- Begin by performing 8 definite, short, fast and strong **squeezes** with your anal sphincter muscle **alternately** with the muscles around and in the penis, as quickly as you can. These should be fast, definite contractions—squeeze and release without holding the contraction. Stay relaxed and focused on the movement.

Bridge Pose: As you exhale, press your feet onto the floor and slowly lift your pelvis off the mat. Raise your hips until your body forms a straight line from your shoulders to your knees, maintaining your pelvis in a neutral position. Hold this bridge for 5 to 10 seconds, ensuring you continue to breathe deeply and steadily throughout.

Release: After the hold, slowly roll your spine back down to the floor, vertebra by vertebra. Once fully lowered, take a deep breath in through your nose, allowing your abdomen to rise. As you exhale slowly, relax your pelvic muscles completely. This deep, abdominal breathing helps release any tension in muscles not under your direct control, promoting full relaxation.

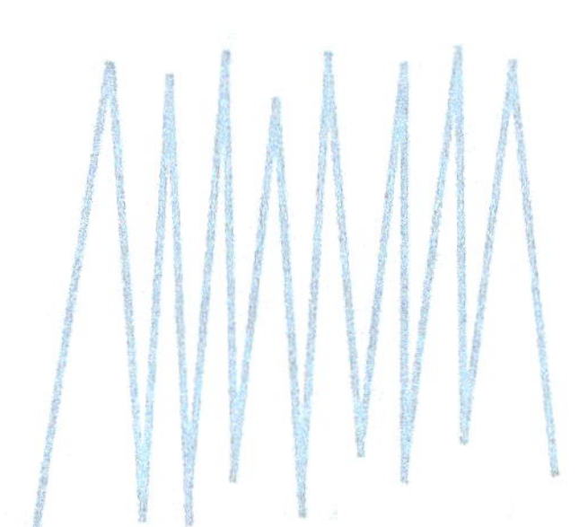

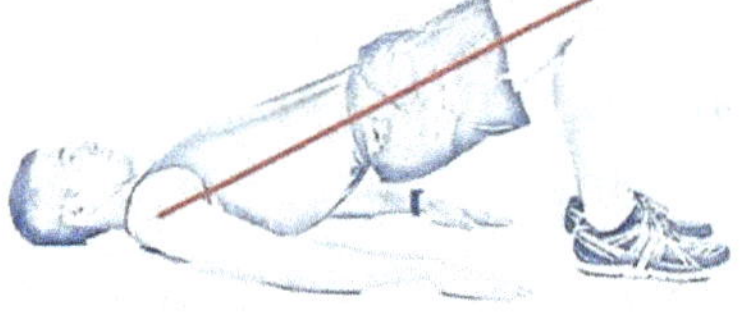

The Total Control Contraction - TCC

What is Total Control Contraction (TCC)?

By this point, you have already gained knowledge on how to engage and relax the musculature surrounding the penis, the anal sphincter, and the region underneath the prostate. The subsequent step is to master the Total Control Contraction (TCC), which entails the simultaneous tightening of all these pelvic floor muscle regions. You will feel all three areas working in unison according to your will; however, the key lies in the conscious control of each zone independently to ensure that every component of the pelvic floor is appropriately engaged. Even before all these three muscle areas were in operation all together; but now the contraction of each section should be checked separately to guarantee that all the pelvic floor muscles are adequately squeezed.

Why is this important? If the pelvic muscles are merely squeezed and relaxed without focus, the stronger muscle (typically the anal sphincter) will dominate, overshadowing the weaker parts of the pelvic floor. Consequently, the weaker areas will not receive the necessary attention for proper muscle development. By **consciously contracting and verifying** each area, you will train all parts of the pelvic floor to grow stronger and more responsive. The Total

Control Contraction (TCC) ensures that all three muscle areas— the muscles around your penis, the anal sphincter, and the muscles beneath the prostate gland should be appropriately squeezed and developed.

Performing the Total Control Contraction (TCC) Exercise

1. **Get into Position**: Start by lying on your back with your **knees bent** and **feet flat on the floor**. Relax your abdominal muscles.

2. **Activate Each Muscle Group**:
   - **First**, perform a squeezing motion as **if you are trying to stop a bowel movement** or control an urgent need to pass gas.
   - Then, engage the muscles **as though you are trying to stop the flow of urine**.
   - Finally, simultaneously try to **"lift" the scrotum up**.

3. **Check Your Contractions**: Mentally check that you are contracting all the three muscle areas and they are fully engaged. Once you are sure each area is squeezed, **relax** the pelvic floor muscles. Let your abdomen soften, and exhale slowly.

Total Control Contraction (TCC) with Maximum Force

The next task is to **perform** a **Total Control Contraction (TCC)** squeeze, engaging your pelvic floor muscles **with maximum force**. This exercise is designed to provide sufficient stimulus to induce muscle growth in the pelvic floor. To achieve this, consciously focus on closing the two openings (anal and urethral) and 'lifting' the scrotum up, pulling it upwards and away from your underwear as much as possible.

After completing the squeeze with maximum force, it's crucial to relax all the three muscle areas fully. When you release your pelvic floor muscles, you should experience a sensation of "letting go," accompanied by a feeling of deep relaxation and rest in the pelvic muscles. This phase of relaxation is just as important as the contraction, allowing your muscles to recover and prevent strain.

Breathing and Muscle Control

Repeat the Exercise and Focus on Breath:
Repeat the **Total Control Contraction (TCC)** squeeze with maximum force, **holding the contraction for a count of 6**. While doing this, pay close attention to your breathing during the squeeze. Ensure that you are breathing naturally and steadily throughout the exercise. Avoid holding your

breath, as this can create unnecessary tension in your body and interfere with the effectiveness of the exercise.

Remember, as you engage your pelvic floor muscles with full intensity, the goal is to challenge them while maintaining proper the squeeze and awareness. Controlled breathing helps you stay relaxed and focused, ensuring that each contraction is both powerful and effective.

Once you have executed the maximum squeeze, ensure that you completely relax each muscle group. As you relax, you should feel a sensation of "letting go," with your pelvic muscles experiencing a deep rest and relaxation.

How did you breathe?

Most of the people holding a strong muscle contraction, are not able to control their breathing. It happens often that during the exhalation phase, they cannot hold the muscle squeeze, and their muscles relax completely or partially, although this is not their intention.

Here is the truth: The pelvic floor muscles are not directly affected by the type of breath you take during exercise. However, to effectively use these muscles in everyday life, it is crucial to learn how to breathe properly while maintaining muscle contractions. Everyday actions like coughing, sneezing, laughing, and talking are all forms of exhalation. While a well-trained strong pelvic floor can manage on its own, there are situations when you will need extra control. For instance, when you have diarrhea or need to hold urine, or to prevent premature ejaculation, maintaining a pelvic muscle squeeze during exhalation is crucial.

Therefore, the goal is not just to strengthen your pelvic floor muscles, but also to learn how to control them under different conditions in everyday life. With practice, you will be able to hold the squeeze during exhalation, ensuring pelvic floor stability when you need it most.

Learning Proper Breathing Technique

As you practice, focus on keeping your attention on your sphincter muscles throughout the exercise. Distraction, even for a moment, can cause the unintentional relaxation of the muscles. During exhalation, your pelvic muscles should remain contracted unless you consciously decide to relax them. A key technique to learn is how to breathe into your chest rather than your abdomen during pelvic floor exercises. When you want to hold a pelvic muscle contraction, **breathe into your chest** rather than your abdomen. If you breathe into your abdomen, then together with the relaxation of the abdominal muscles, also your sphincter muscle will be relaxed. Don't worry if this doesn't come naturally at first. With regular practice, you will be able to hold the pelvic floor contraction even during exhalation.

Tricky Exercise to Demonstrate How to Use Your Pelvic Floor Muscles in Daily Life

The following exercise will help you **automatically engage** your pelvic floor muscles in everyday situations.

! When you perform the Total Control squeeze, you should always focus on your weaker sphincter muscle, contracting it with maximum force. This ensures that both your stronger and weaker sphincter muscles will be tightened correctly. By practicing this regularly, you will be able to maintain pelvic muscle control during normal activities like coughing, sneezing, delaying ejaculation or holding in urine when a restroom is not immediately available.

In supine position with knees bent, feet flat on the floor. Start with a few abdominal breathings. During the inhalation phase, you should feel as your belly expand comfortably,

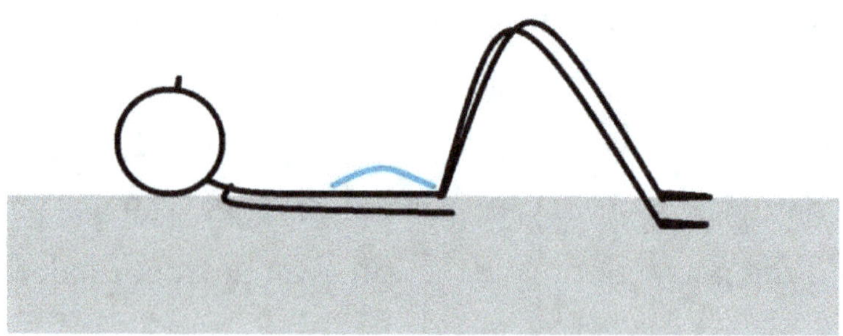

As you exhale press your knees against each other, perform a **Total Control Contraction** (**TCC**) with maximum force, as you exhale next, holding the squeeze, lift your hips off the mat, still holding the squeeze, slowly lower your hips to the starting position,

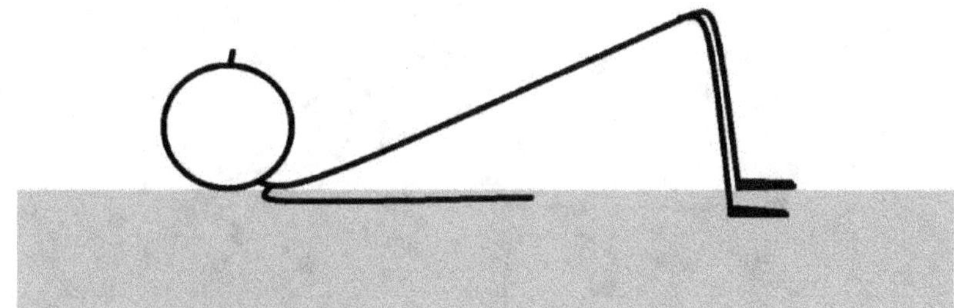

Still holding the **Total Control Contraction**, raise your trunk up off the floor, roll back and relax. During the next inhalation phase, you should feel as your belly expand comfortably,

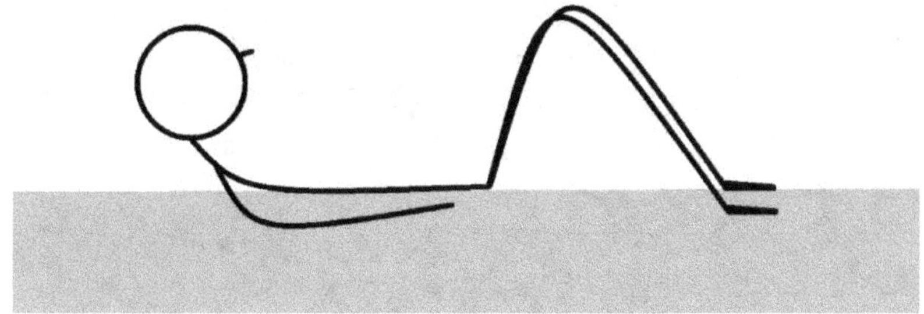

As you exhale perform a **Total Control** squeeze with maximum force, holding the contraction, begin to open up your knees apart, but only up to that point, where still you can hold the squeeze of the pelvic floor muscles, keep your legs in this position, begin to "waving" with your legs slightly apart 4 times ("little openings"),

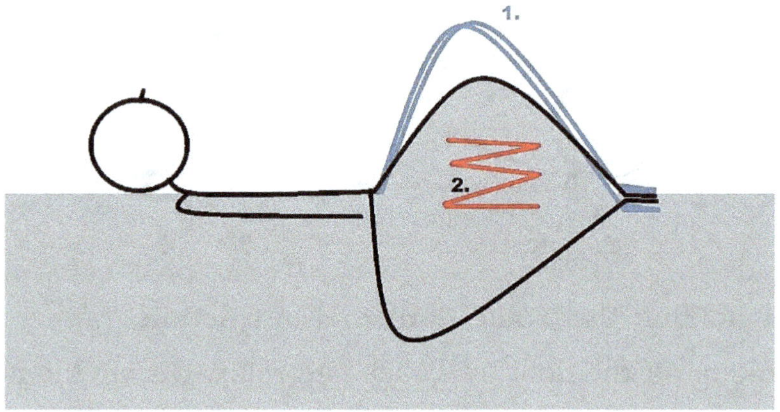

As you exhale, close your knees pressing against each other, during the next exhalation phase lift your hips off the mat,

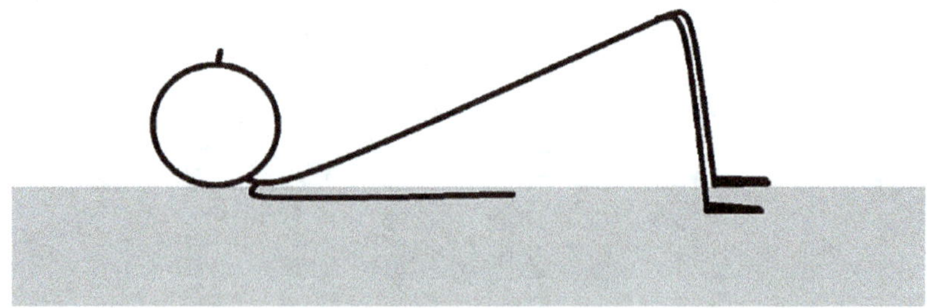

Still holding the **Total Control** squeeze, slowly lower your hips to the starting position, and relax your muscles, spread your knees as far apart as possible, let your abdominal muscles become soft, slow elongated exhalation. Perform 3-4 abdominal breathing.

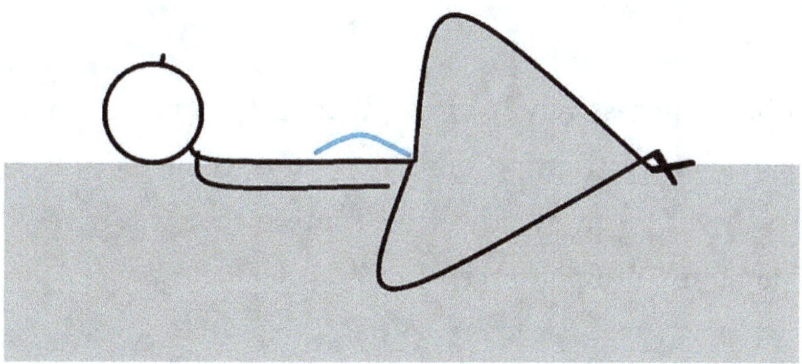

Have you been able to finish the entire exercise?

If not, don't worry, this exercise requires strong and well-trained pelvic muscles. Keep practicing, and over time, you will build the strength and control needed to hold these contractions for longer periods, in any situation.

Note: Once you can **maintain a contraction** in supine position (while lying down), you will gradually be able to do it in other postures and situations—walking, standing, or even during sexual intercourse. This training prepares your pelvic muscles for spontaneous use during activities like sneezing, coughing, or when you are unable to reach a restroom quickly.

Congratulations! You have Mastered the Basics—Now Let's Level Up!

You have successfully learned the foundational movements of pelvic floor training, and now it is time to challenge yourself with a more advanced routine that will take your pelvic floor strength to the next level.

Chapter 4: Advanced Pelvic Health Routines for Everyday Life

Advanced Workout Plan To The Everyday Practice

Functional Fitness and Everyday Movement with a Strong Pelvic Floor

This is where the real magic happens. Strengthening your pelvic floor isn't just about improving in the gym—it enhances your daily life. Whether it is lifting heavy objects, running after your kids, or simply running, a strong pelvic floor makes everything smoother and safer. That is what functional fitness is all about—building strength that benefits your everyday movements. For the first few weeks, I recommend starting with this advanced pelvic floor workout to strengthen your muscles. Once your pelvic floor muscles are strong, you can perform these exercises and combine them as you see fit. The beauty of pelvic floor exercises is that you can practice them in any position that feels comfortable—whether you are lying down, sitting, standing, or even during your daily activities.

Balance scale exercise with pelvic tilt:

Part A: In supine position with knees bent, feet flat the floor (close to each other). Relax your abdominal muscles. Pay attention only to the muscles around and in your penis. Squeeze the muscles around your penis, just a little bit, hold this slight tension. Move your pelvis forward, in this position there is a small "bridge" under the lower back. Increase the force of the contraction of the muscles around and in your penis until your maximum force; squeeze your penis tightly, try to "lift" the scrotum up as high as you can, "pull back" the base of your penis toward the rectum. Hold the squeeze counting to 6; squeeze the penis in its full-length. As you exhale, slowly, counting to 4, relax your penis muscles. Let your abdominal muscles become soft, perform a slow elongated exhalation. Allow the spine and pelvis to return to their original – neutral position.

Before continuing the exercise, take a break counting to 5.

Part B: Relax your abdominal muscles. Pay attention only to the sphincter muscle ring around your anus. Squeeze slightly the muscles around the anus, hold this slight tension, move your pelvis backward – simultaneously tighten your buttock muscles and press your lower back down into the mat, increase the force of contraction of your buttock till the maximum force, squeeze the muscles around the anus as strongly as you can. Hold the squeeze counting to 6. As you exhale, slowly, counting to 4 relax your muscles. Let your abdominal muscles become soft, make a slow elongated exhalation, almost like a sigh of relief. Allow the spine and pelvis to return to their original – neutral position. Before repeating the **Part A** exercise, take a break counting to 5.

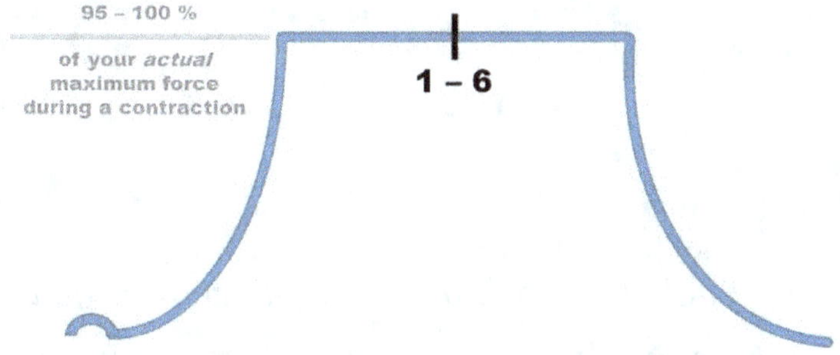

At the end of the repetitions of the exercise **(Part A-B), one time**, perform 8 definite, short, fast and strong contractions **alternately** with your muscles around and in the penis and anal sphincter muscle, as quickly as you can. Do not try to hold the contractions, just squeeze and relax. Remain in supine position, with knees bent. In order to maintain a balance, place your arms on the floor alongside your body, palms facing down. As you exhale press your feet onto the floor, slowly lift your pelvis up off the mat into a bridge, your pelvis is in line with your shoulders and knees; hold this position for 5 to 10 seconds. Remember to breathe! Release and roll slowly back down to the floor. Inhale deeply through your nose into your abdomen and slowly blow out the air while you relax your pelvis completely.

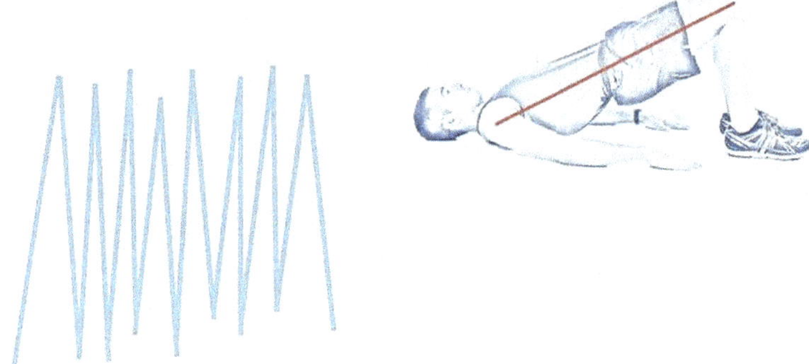

If you cannot hold this position, as an alternative you can place a cushion under your buttocks to keep them raised

In the first 2 weeks:

Hold the squeeze for a count of 6 and before you pass to the B part of the exercise take a break for a count of 5.

Before repeating the exercise (Part A), take a break counting to 5. Repeat the exercise 3 times.

Between 2 - 4 weeks:

Hold the squeeze for a count of 8 and before you pass to the B part of the exercise take a break for a count of 5.

Before repeating the exercise (Part A), take a break counting to 5. Repeat the exercise 5 times.

After 4 weeks:

Hold the squeeze for a count of 10 and before you pass to the B part of the exercise take a break for a count of 5.

Before repeating the exercise (Part A), take a break counting to 5. Repeat the exercise 5 times.

"Bow Tie" exercise:

Sit in "Z" leg position (the legs make the shape of a letter "Z"); the left knee pulled up in front and the right heel pulled back. Relax your abdominal muscles.

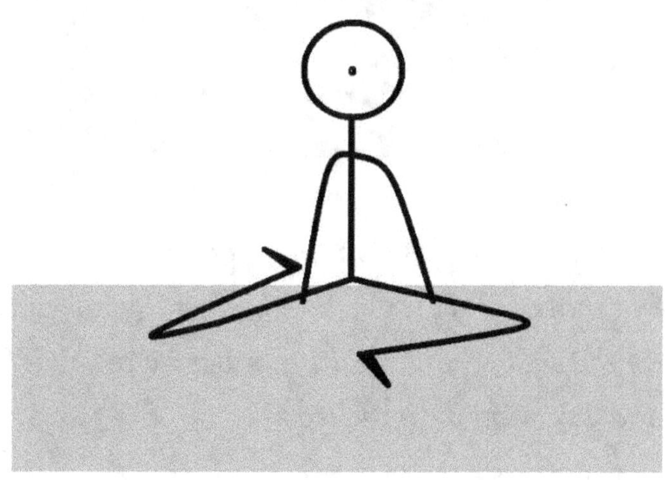

If you are not able to settle yourself in this Z-leg position you can sit in a butterfly position.

Sit with the soles of your feet together, so in this position your knees point out to the sides. Grab your legs with your hands.

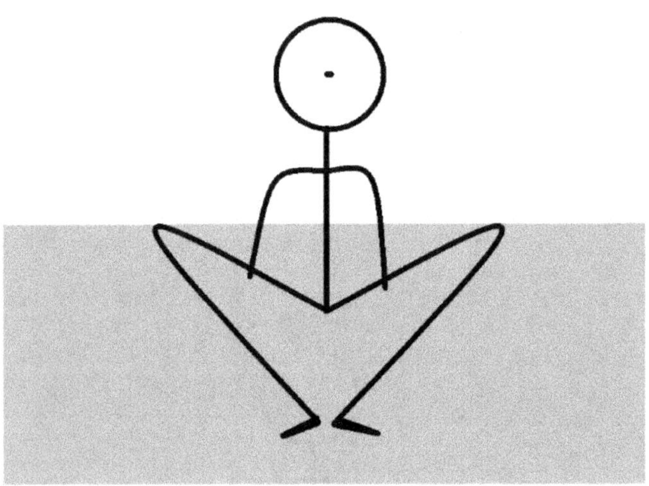

Another alternative position, open your legs wide as you can, in the shape of the letter V, then, bend your right knee and place the sole of your right foot beside to the left knee, change the direction with the legs.

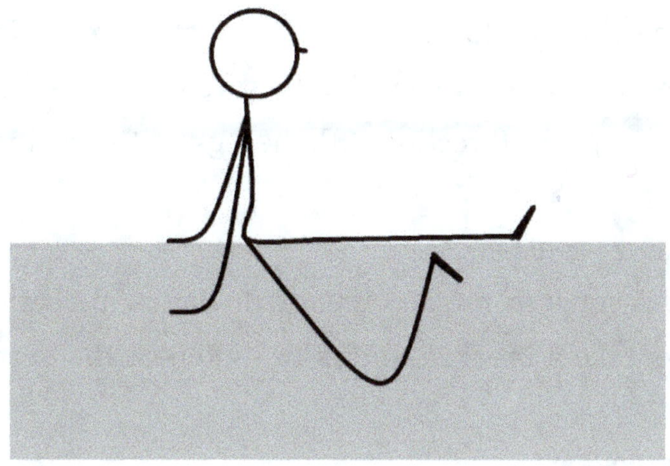

The task is to perform gradually a Total Control squeeze, counting to 4, hold the squeeze for a count of 6, without relaxing the muscles completely, immediately perform 4 Total Control contractions, as quickly as you can, increase again the strength of the contraction till your maximum force and at the end counting to 4, gradually let your pelvic floor muscles completely relax. Before repeating the exercise, **take a break** counting to 5.

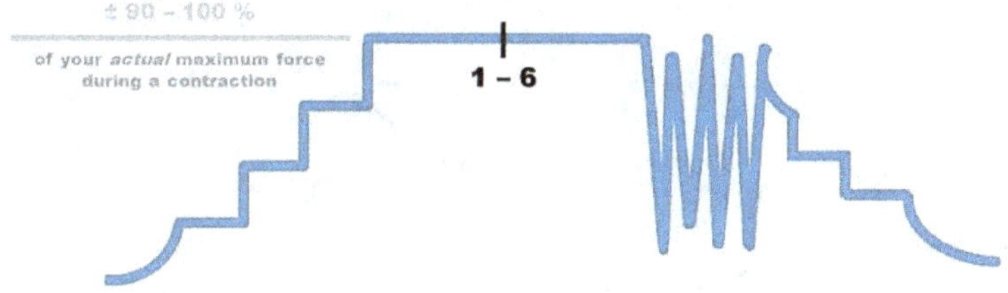

In the first 2 weeks:

Hold the squeeze for a count of 6. Before repeating the exercise, take a break counting to 5. Repeat the exercise 3 times. Change the direction with the legs (in the position 1 or 3)

Between 2 - 4 weeks:

Hold the squeeze for a count of 8. Before repeating the exercise, take a break counting to 5. Repeat the exercise 3 times.

After 4 weeks:

Hold the squeeze for a count of 12. Before repeating the exercise, take a break counting to 15. Repeat the exercise 3 times.

Penis power exercise:

In supine position with knees bent, feet flat on the floor. Feet and knees are in hip distance apart.

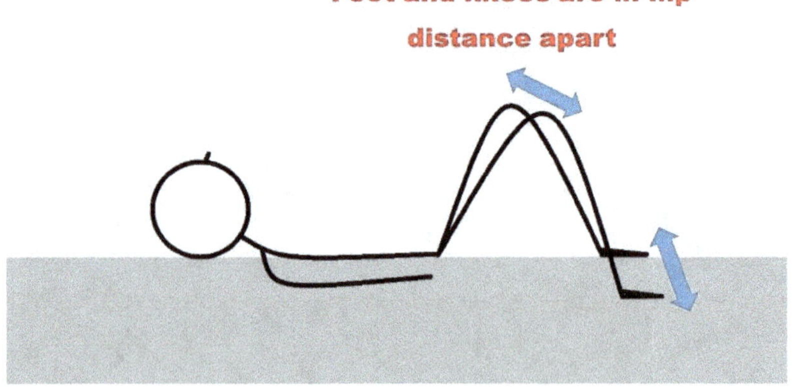

The task is to perform suddenly a contraction with the muscles around and in the penis, up to the 50% of the maximum strength, right after increase the force of the squeeze, up to your maximum force, then perform 4 short and fast contractions but releasing back the strength of the squeeze only up to the 50 % of your maximum force, after increase again and hold the squeeze on the maximum strength, counting to 6. Release the contraction of the muscles back only up to the 50 % of your maximum force - hold the squeeze at 50% counting to 4 at the and gradually let the muscles relax completely. Exhale slowly.

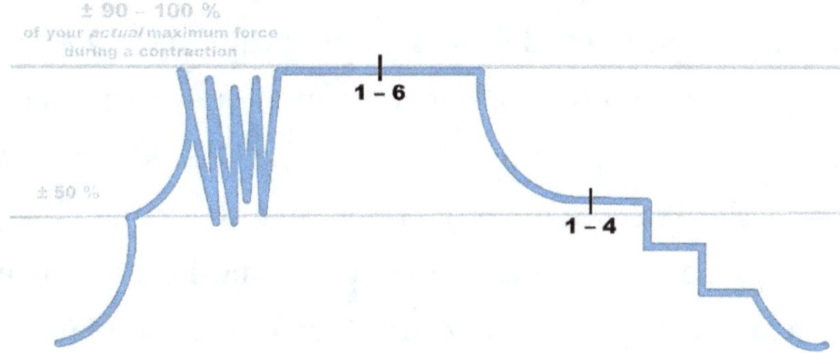

In the first 2 weeks:

Hold the squeeze at the maximum force for a count of 6 and on the 50% of the maximum force counting to 4. Before repeating the exercise, take a break counting to 10. Repeat the exercise 3 times.

Between 2-4 weeks:

Hold the squeeze at the maximum force for a count of 8 and on the 50% of the maximum force counting to 6. Before repeating the exercise, take a break counting to 10. Repeat the exercise 3 times.

After 4 weeks:

Hold the squeeze at the maximum force for a count of 10 and on the 50% of the maximum force counting to 10. Before repeating the exercise, take a break counting to 20. Repeat the exercise 3 times.

At the end of the repetitions of the exercise, **one time**, perform 8 definite, short, fast and strong contractions with the muscles around and in your penis; as quickly as you can. Do not try to hold the contractions; just squeeze and relax. Remain in supine position, with knees bent. Feet and knees are very close to each other or closed. In order to maintain a balance, place your arms on the floor alongside your body, palms facing down. As you exhale press your feet onto the floor, slowly lift your pelvis up off the mat into a bridge, your pelvis is in line with your shoulders and knees, hold this position for 5 to 10 seconds. Remember to breathe! Release and roll slowly back down to the floor. Inhale deeply through your nose into your abdomen and slowly blow out the air while you relax your pelvis completely.

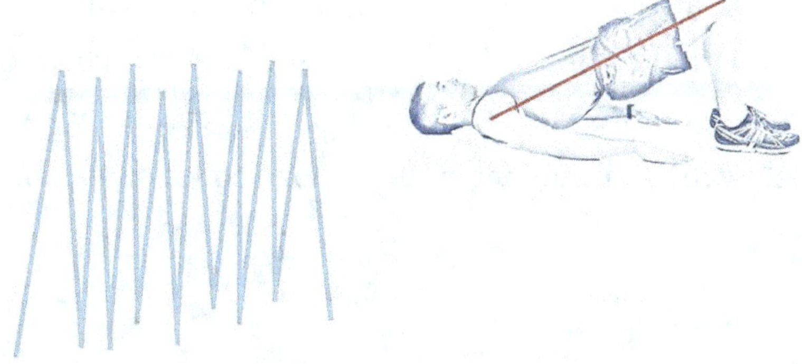

Exercise to strengthen the anal sphincter:

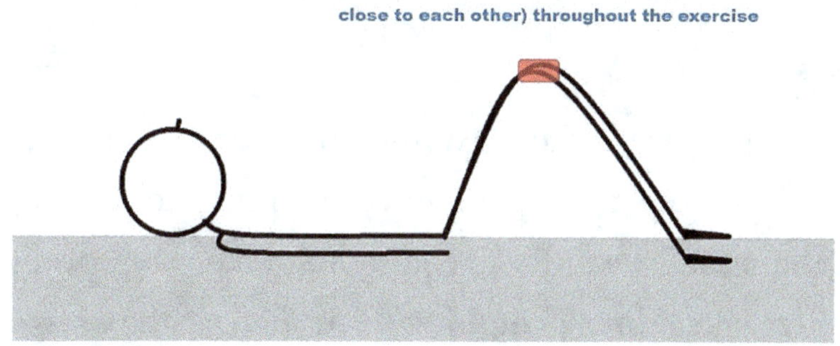

In supine position, keep the feet and knees together or very close to each other.

The task is, while counting to 4, gradually squeeze the anal sphincter muscle to the maximum strength, hold the contraction at 100% for a count of 4, relax back the muscles around the anus to 50% of the maximum strength, and hold the squeeze at 50% for a count of 4, increase the strength of the contraction again to the maximum force, and keep the squeeze at 100% for a count of 4, finally gradually relax completely the anal sphincter muscle for a count of 4. Exhale slowly.

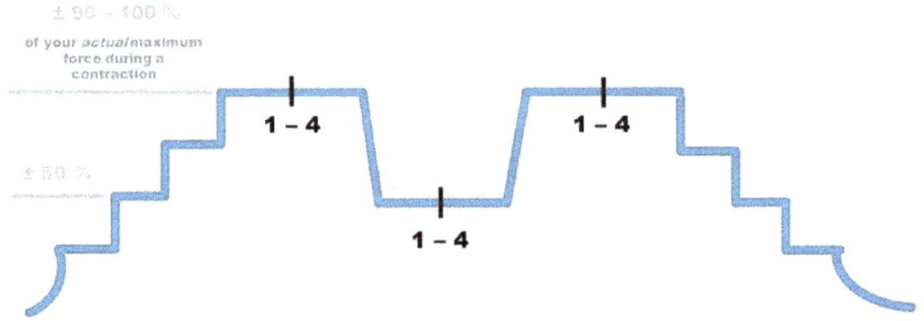

In the first 2 weeks:

Hold the squeeze at the maximum force for a count of 4 - on the 50% of the maximum force counting to 4 - at the maximum force again for a count of 4. Before repeating the exercise, take a break counting to 10. Repeat the exercise 3 times.

Between 2-4 weeks:

Hold the squeeze at the maximum force for a count of 6 - on the 50% of the maximum force counting to 6 - at the maximum force again for a count of 6. Before repeating the exercise, take a break counting to 10. Repeat the exercise 3 times.

__After 4 weeks:__

Hold the squeeze at the maximum force for a count of 10 - on the 50% of the maximum force counting to 6 - at the maximum force again for a count of 10. Before repeating the exercise, take a break counting to 15. Repeat the exercise 3 times.

At the end of the repetition of the exercise, **one time**, perform 8 definite, short, fast and strong contractions with the anal sphincter muscle, as quickly as you can. Do not try to hold the contractions, just squeeze and relax. Remain in supine position, with knees bent. Feet and knees are very close to each other or closed. In order to maintain a balance, place your arms on the floor alongside your body, palms facing down. As you exhale press your feet onto the floor, slowly lift your pelvis up off the mat into a bridge, your pelvis is in line with your shoulders and knees; hold this position for 10 seconds. Remember to breathe! Release and roll slowly back down to the floor. Inhale deeply through your nose into your abdomen and slowly blow out the air while you relax your pelvis completely.

Total pelvic power exercise

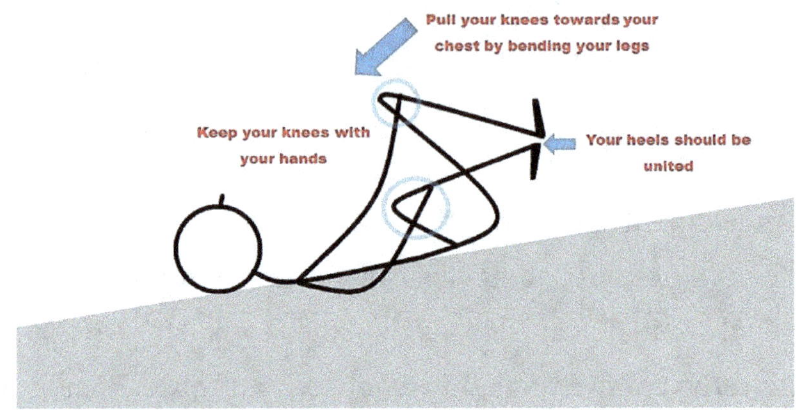

Lying position. Pull both knees toward your chest by flexing your legs. Keep your knees with your hands. Your heels should be united.

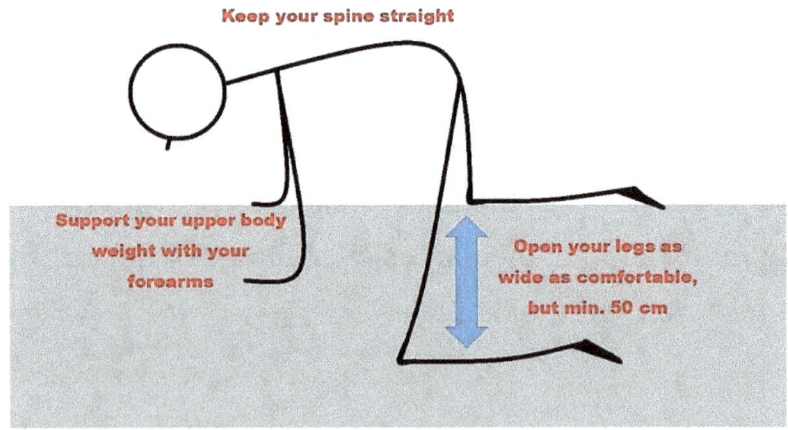

In "all fours" position. Support your upper - body weight with your forearms. Keep your spine straight. Open your legs as wide as comfortable but min. should be 50 cm.

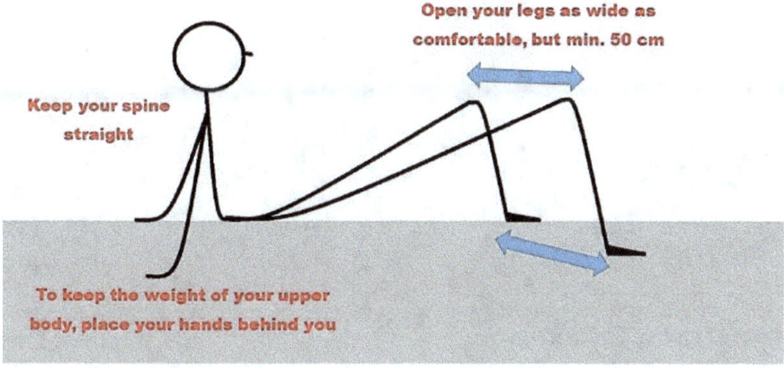

In sitting position with knees bent. Keep your spine straight. Support your upper body with your hands. Spread your legs as wide apart as you can.

The task is to perform suddenly a Total Control squeeze up to the maximum force, hold the squeeze for a count of 6, then gradually counting to 4, let the pelvic floor muscles to relax almost completely, right after quickly perform 6 Total Control squeeze as fast as you can, without a pause, make suddenly a Total Control contraction again, up to the 50 % of your maximum force, hold the squeeze for a count of 4, at the end let your pelvic floor muscles to relax completely.

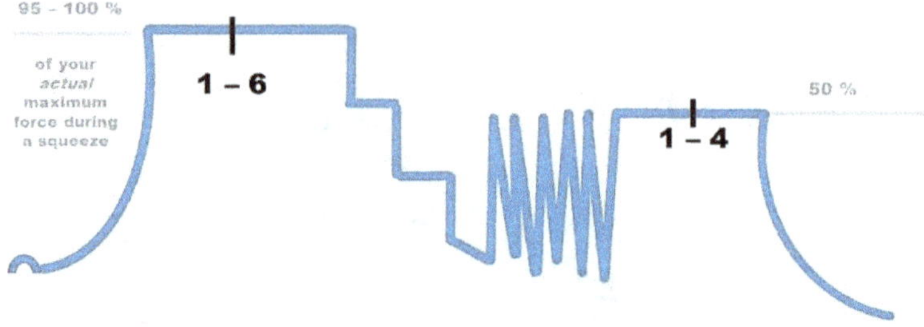

In the first 4 weeks:

Hold the squeeze at the maximum of your force as you count to 6 - on 50% of the maximum strength counting to 4. Before repeating the exercise, take a break counting to 10. Repeat the exercise 2 times in each posture.

After 4 weeks:

Hold the squeeze at the maximum force for a count of 10 - on the 50% of the maximum force counting to 10. Before repeating the exercise, take a break counting to 30. Repeat the exercise 2 times in each posture.

How to Fit Pelvic Floor Exercises into Your Busy Day

Maintaining pelvic health is not a one-time effort but a lifelong commitment. The key to lasting benefits lies in building sustainable habits, seamlessly integrating exercises into your daily life, and effectively addressing any setbacks you may encounter. You might be wondering, how do I fit these exercises into my already busy schedule? Here is the beauty of pelvic floor exercises: they can be done almost anywhere and don't require any equipment. You can discreetly engage your pelvic floor muscles without anyone knowing. Whether you are stuck in traffic, brushing your teeth, or even watching Netflix, you can engage your pelvic floor without anyone noticing. Making pelvic floor exercises a regular part of your routine doesn't have to feel like a burden. Another tip? Pair the exercises with something you already do every day. Also, you can use technology to your advantage. Set reminders on your phone or calendar to prompt you when it's time for your pelvic exercises. Here is an example of how to make it part of your routine:

Morning Routine:
In the morning, before you even get out of bed, do your first set of ten basic Kegels. Make a few contractions, holding each for five to ten seconds, and then resting for five seconds. Or, if you're feeling confident, choose your favorite exercise

from the advanced Kegel workout and repeat it 2–5 times, as you prefer. Maybe you have a morning coffee or tea ritual. Why not add your pelvic floor routine to that time? The key is to link these exercises to something you already enjoy so they don't slip off your radar and they become a natural part of your day, not an extra task.

Afternoon Breaks:

In the afternoon, do a few Kegels while you are sitting at your desk, taking a lunch break, or waiting in line at the grocery store. It's fun knowing that others have no idea what you're doing! These little moments add up over time, helping reinforce your pelvic strength.

Evening Routine:

Finally, in the evening, mix in some pelvic tilts or bridges as part of your regular workout. These exercises are fantastic for engaging in the lower core and pelvic muscles. Or, put your newly strengthened pelvic floor muscles to use in the bedroom, enhancing both your pleasure and your partner's. The benefits of a strong pelvic floor go far beyond just exercise, they can enrich your intimate life as well.

Pelvic Floor Exercises for Enhanced Sexual Health

By now, it should be clear that your pelvic floor muscles are far more important than you might have initially realized. They play a central role in sexual satisfaction:

- **For Women:** Strong pelvic floor muscles enhance orgasm intensity and make achieving orgasms easier.
- **For Men:** These muscles play a key role in improving erections and helping them last longer in bed.

Once you have mastered this advanced Kegel workout, you can even surprise your partner during sex. Yes, **during sex!** You can delay your orgasm and prolong sexual intercourse, which will take your intimacy to the next level. You can repeat the stop-squeeze technique several times, pausing for a few seconds, or you can do it once. (Total Control contraction: keep the contraction for 3-5 seconds then relax the muscles). Be intuitive, experiment, and create your own repertoire. I guarantee your partner will notice—and love—the difference!

Building a Routine That Fits Your Life

That's it—a simple routine that only takes a few minutes each day but can deliver significant results over time. As you get more comfortable with the exercises, start increasing the length of time you hold each Kegel and the number of repetitions in each session. Combining core and pelvic floor exercises is one of the best things you can do for your overall strength, stability, and health.

- **Posture Improvement:** These exercises will enhance your posture, reducing back and hip pain.

- **Better Body Control:** You will gain greater control over your body, both in everyday life and in the bedroom.

- **Confidence from Within:** Remember, it is not just about looking good (though that's a nice bonus). It's about feeling strong, confident, and in control—from the inside out.

Make It a Habit, Not a Chore

The key is to make pelvic floor exercises feel easy to fit into your life as an enjoyable part of your routine. You don't need to dedicate an hour each day to them—small sessions sprinkled throughout the day are more than enough to see progress. A few minutes here and there can make all the difference.

Stay Motivated with Realistic Goals

And let's not forget the importance of setting realistic goals. Keep your motivation high by reminding yourself of the benefits of a strong pelvic floor. Recognize that building muscle strength, particularly in the pelvic floor, is a gradual process. It may take weeks or even months before you notice significant improvements. One of the biggest motivation killers is expecting immediate results. You will not see massive changes overnight, but small, consistent progress is the sweet spot. Celebrate the little victories along the way:

- **Did you notice better bladder control this week?** Awesome!
- **Were you able to last longer in bed?** Fantastic!

These small wins will keep you motivated. Remember, pelvic floor health is not just about solving problems, it's about maximizing your potential and living your best life. Long-term pelvic health requires commitment, creativity, and a sense of humor.

So, take that first step, and before you know it, you will be the master of your pelvic floor—and by extension, your health, confidence, and vitality.

Lifestyle Habits that Impact Pelvic Floor Health

Our pelvic floor muscles are like hidden heroes, silently supporting us in so many ways throughout the day—whether we are sitting at our desks, lifting groceries, or even laughing with friends. The strength and health of these muscles are shaped not just by exercises like Kegels but also by the small, everyday habits we may not even think about. Understanding how certain lifestyle habits can either support or weaken your pelvic floor helps ensure long-lasting sexual vitality, optimal wellness, and sexual confidence. From what we eat and drink to how we manage stress, these simple routines can make a world of difference when it comes to our pelvic health. This chapter will guide you through practical tips on how to care about your pelvic floor, starting with something as simple as your diet and ending with essential hygiene routines.

Diet and Hydration: Fueling Your Pelvic Floor

You are what you eat—this saying holds especially true when it comes to your pelvic floor health. Just like any other muscle in your body, your pelvic floor depends on good nutrition to stay strong and functional. What you eat and drink directly affects how well these muscles perform, and in some cases, the wrong choices can lead to issues like constipation, bladder irritation, and pelvic floor strain. Let's look at how you can support your pelvic floor through thoughtful dietary choices.

Hydration: A Key to Pelvic Health

Staying well-hydrated is crucial not only for your overall health but also for maintaining a strong pelvic floor. Dehydration can lead to constipation, which forces you to strain during bowel movements, weakening the pelvic muscles over time. Drinking plenty of water helps keep your stool soft, making bowel movements easier and preventing unnecessary strain.

However, balance is the key—drinking too much water can overfill your bladder, causing frequent urination and potentially weakening the pelvic floor. Some men cut back on liquids in an effort to reduce frequent urination or leakage, but this strategy backfires. Your body needs adequate water to function properly, and staying hydrated also helps flush out toxins, keeping your urinary system healthy.

Dehydration doesn't just lead to constipation; it can also cause fatigue, headaches, and urinary issues. Drinking enough water ensures that your bladder empties fully, which reduces the risk of urinary tract infections. When dealing with conditions like cystitis and prostatitis, increasing your fluid intake is particularly important to help clear the bladder.

So, what is the golden rule? Drink enough water so your urine is a light-yellow color. Too little water can result in concentrated urine that irritates your bladder and prostate, while too much water can cause frequent bathroom trips that overwork your pelvic muscles. As always, moderation is key.

Foods That Strengthen the Pelvic Muscles

The pelvic floor is part of a larger system, and when this system is well-nourished, everything functions more smoothly. Including the right foods in your diet can promote not only pelvic health but also overall muscle strength.

- **Fiber-Rich Foods**: If you have ever had to deal with constipation, you know how much it can strain your body—and your pelvic floor isn't exempt from that stress. A diet rich in fiber from whole grains, fruits, vegetables, and legumes helps keep things moving, which reduces the need for straining during bowel movements. However, remember, fiber needs a partner: **water**. Drinking plenty of fluids ensures that fiber can do its job effectively. Otherwise, an increase in fiber without enough hydration could actually make things worse.

- **Lean Proteins**: Protein is essential for muscle repair and strength, and your pelvic floor is no exception. Including lean meats, fish, eggs, and plant-based proteins like beans and lentils in your diet will help maintain your pelvic floor's resilience. However, it is wise to moderate your intake of meat—especially processed or hormone-treated cuts—since these can affect your hormone balance. Opt for plant-based meals whenever possible to keep things in check.

- **Healthy Fats**: Omega-3 fatty acids, found in fish, nuts, and seeds, are known to reduce inflammation, which can otherwise contribute to pelvic floor weakness. In addition, these healthy fats support overall muscle function and tissue repair, helping your body bounce back from wear and tear.

Foods to Avoid

Just as certain foods can support your pelvic floor, others can irritate it or make it harder for your muscles to function properly. Being mindful of these foods and drinks will help you avoid unnecessary strain.

Caffeine and alcohol: Both act as diuretics, which increase the frequency of urination and put unnecessary strain on your bladder and pelvic floor. Limiting your intake of coffee, tea, and alcoholic beverages can help reduce pressure on your pelvic muscles and improve overall bladder control.

Spicy and acidic foods: These can irritate the bladder lining, potentially worsening incontinence, prostatitis or causing discomfort. If you notice bladder sensitivity after consuming foods like tomatoes, citrus fruits, or spicy dishes, it might be time to cut back or eliminate them from your diet to prevent irritation.

Processed foods: Highly processed foods often lack the fiber necessary for healthy digestion, which can lead to constipation and increased straining during bowel movements, both of which weaken the pelvic floor over time. In addition, excessive sugar and unhealthy fats in these foods can contribute to inflammation and poor muscle function, including in your pelvic floor. Opting for a more natural, fiber-rich diet can keep your digestive system functioning smoothly and support your pelvic health.

Supplements for Pelvic Health

If you are looking to go beyond, there are supplements that can support your pelvic floor health.

Magnesium is a mineral often recommended for overall muscle health, including the pelvic floor, as it helps relax muscles and prevent cramping. It can also relieve constipation, which benefits your pelvic floor by reducing strain during bowel movements.

Electrolytes are essential for fluid balance in the body, supporting both muscle and nerve function. They also aid in muscle repair, which is crucial after workouts or heavy movements.

Omega-3 fatty acids, found for example in fish oil or flaxseed, reduce inflammation and promote healthy muscle function. These can be especially helpful if you are dealing with pelvic floor discomfort or stiffness.

Vitamin C is a powerful antioxidant and immune booster that helps your body fight off infections like cystitis, which can affect the bladder and pelvic floor muscles.

Probiotics are great for maintaining a healthy balance of intestinal flora. A healthy gut can support overall health by keeping your immune system strong and your digestion functioning smoothly, which also reduces the risk of infections.

Zinc is one of the most important trace minerals in human nutrition, and its deficiency is a widespread problem. Zinc plays a role in tissue repair and immune function, so it can also support the health of your pelvic floor.

Turmeric is another great supplement to consider. Known for its anti-inflammatory, antioxidant, and even anticancer properties, turmeric can help fight bacterial and viral infections, improving prostate and bladder health. For those dealing with cystitis or prostatitis, taking 1000 mg of pure turmeric capsules daily for at least 30 days might help. However, turmeric is not for everyone—avoid it if you have gallstones, bile duct issues, or if you are on blood-thinning medications.

There is also a helpful *herbal remedy*: birch leaf tea. This natural ally for bladder health is known for increasing urine production, which can help clear out the urinary tract and even dissolve kidney stones, allowing the body to expel them painlessly. To make it, boil two tablespoons of dried birch leaves in half a liter of water, let it sit for 10-15 minutes, strain, and drink the tea within 30 minutes—preferably in the morning. Don't forget to drink a lot of water throughout the day to flush out toxins, bacteria or whatever harmful things from your body! Repeat this cleanse once or twice a week. However, if you are allergic to aspirin, avoid birch tea, as it contains salicylates.

Just remember, don't go overboard with supplements. Start with the basics, and if you ever have questions, your pharmacist can guide you on how to integrate these supplements safely into your routine.

Manage Stress and Stay Active

Stress is sneaky. It doesn't just affect your mood or sleep—it shows up physically, and for many men, it manifests in the pelvic floor. When you are under constant stress, your body enters fight-or-flight mode, causing muscles throughout your body—including your pelvic floor—to tense up. Over time, this can lead to pelvic floor dysfunction, where the muscles either become overly tight and painful or, in some cases, too weak from being overworked due to constant tension.

You might be thinking, "Well, I can't just stop being stressed." And you're right, life is stressful, and trying to eliminate stress entirely is impossible. However, managing how you respond to stress can make a huge difference in protecting your pelvic floor and overall health.

So, what is the real secret weapon? Exercise. Physical activity is one of the best stress-busters out there. Regular exercise helps release tension and improves your mood, which in turn reduces the strain on your pelvic floor. However, balance is key. While physical activity helps manage stress, overdoing it with exhaustive workouts can temporarily disrupt hormone levels, leading to even more stress on your body. Finding that balance is crucial for both your mental and physical health.

Prioritize Sleep and Recovery

Sleep is crucial for maintaining healthy hormone levels, which directly influences pelvic health. Skimping on sleep, even by just a few hours, can disrupt your hormone balance and increase the risk of pelvic floor issues. Aim for 7-8 hours of quality sleep each night to allow your body to recover and recharge, ensuring proper hormone regulation and muscle repair.

Avoiding Harmful Habits

Certain lifestyle habits, whether related to posture, smoking, or even the clothes we wear—can put unnecessary strain on the pelvic floor. By addressing these habits, you can protect your muscles and maintain pelvic health for years to come.

Smoking and Its Impact

Smoking is particularly harmful to the pelvic floor for two main reasons. First, nicotine constricts blood vessels, reducing blood flow to the pelvic region. Without adequate circulation, the muscles and tissues weaken over time. Second, smoking often leads to chronic coughing, which repeatedly stresses the pelvic floor muscles. Men who smoke are at a much higher risk of developing incontinence due to this constant strain. To protect yourself, try engaging your pelvic floor muscles as you cough or sneeze. This small action can help stabilize your bladder and reduce pressure on the supporting ligaments.

Be Mindful of Toxins and Steer Clear of Harmful Substances

Environmental pollutants and toxins can burden your body's detoxification systems and disrupt hormonal balance. Regular detoxification practices, such as consuming herbal teas or intermittent fasting, can support your body in clearing out harmful substances. A simple way to start is by incorporating a one-day detox each week, focusing on nutrient-rich fruits and vegetables to help cleanse your body and your lymphatic system.

Fitness and Exercise: Moving with Purpose

Physical activity is vital for keeping your whole body, including your pelvic floor, in good shape. But did you know that some types of exercise can actually weaken these muscles if done improperly? Understanding how different movements affect your pelvic floor can help you tailor your fitness routine to protect and strengthen these important muscles.

Core Strengthening for Pelvic Health

Your pelvic floor and core muscles work closely together to provide stability and strength, so focusing on core exercises can be incredibly beneficial. Workouts that engage your deep abdominal muscles or the muscles located in the lower back, like Pilates, yoga and swimming help not only with posture but also with pelvic floor function.

- **Pilates**: This method is excellent for building core strength while being mindful of the pelvic floor. Movements like pelvic tilts and bridges are especially good at activating these muscles without putting too much pressure on them.
- **Yoga**: Many yoga poses naturally engage the pelvic floor. For example, Child's Pose and Bridge Pose help gently strengthen the muscles while also encouraging relaxation and flexibility. Yoga also emphasizes deep, controlled breathing, which can ease tension in your pelvic region.
- **Swimming**, too, is a gentle form of exercise that promotes overall muscle strength, and it avoids the high impact on your pelvic muscles that you might get from running or weightlifting.

Avoiding Harmful Movements

While exercise is important, not all-physical activity is pelvic floor friendly. Heavy lifting, for example, can strain the pelvic muscles, especially if you are not using the correct technique. Always engage your core muscles and exhale during lifting to minimize pressure on your pelvic floor. If your muscles aren't strong enough to handle certain activities, consider building up your strength first before attempting more strenuous exercises.

And here's an important tip: before you lift anything heavy—whether it's weights at the gym or just a bag of groceries—make sure your bladder is empty. A full bladder under pressure can stretch the ligaments that support your pelvic organs, which can lead to long-term damage.

Let's see how to practice different sport activities in the right way.

Jumping and Aerobics: When you engage in activities that involve jumping, such as skipping or high-impact aerobics, your internal organs are also "jumping." This places extra pressure on the supporting ligaments of the pelvic organs, especially overtime. For this reason, it's best to limit these kinds of exercises or, at the very least, approach them mindfully. Low-impact alternatives like fast-paced walking can be just as effective without the added strain on the pelvic floor.

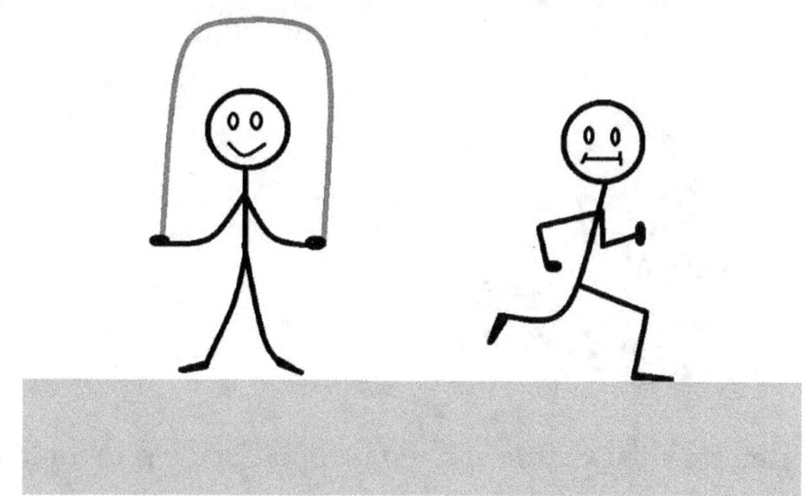

Running: If running is your passion, great! Just make sure to protect yourself with the right posture and equipment. Good running shoes are essential to cushion each step and reduce the impact on your pelvic organs. Also, focus on strengthening your pelvic floor muscles through targeted exercises. Running with poor technique or inadequate support can lead to damage in both the pelvic floor and lower back. If you run, try to land softly and avoid strong jolts while running. If you want to avoid stress on your pelvic floor, consider walking or elliptical training. These exercises are gentler on your pelvic muscles while still providing cardiovascular benefits.

Swimming: Swimming is generally a fantastic exercise, but it is not without its precautions. Always dry yourself properly after water sport activities and change into dry clothes, as wet clothes may cause urinary tract infections.

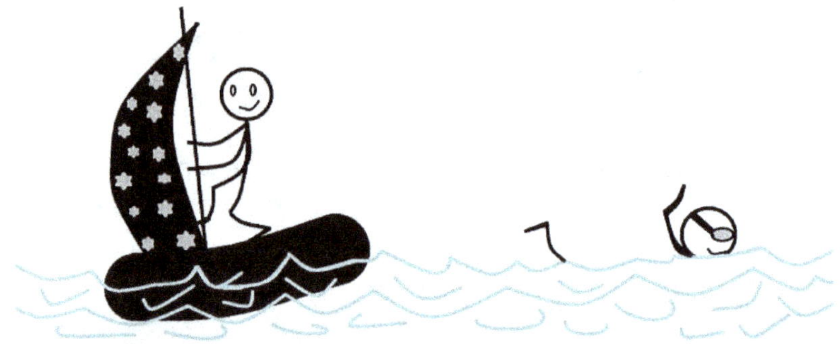

Stretching with Caution: Exercises that involve a straddle position—legs wide apart—can put stress on the pelvic area. To minimize strain, always engage your pelvic floor muscles during these movements. This helps to protect your pelvic organs and prevent injury.

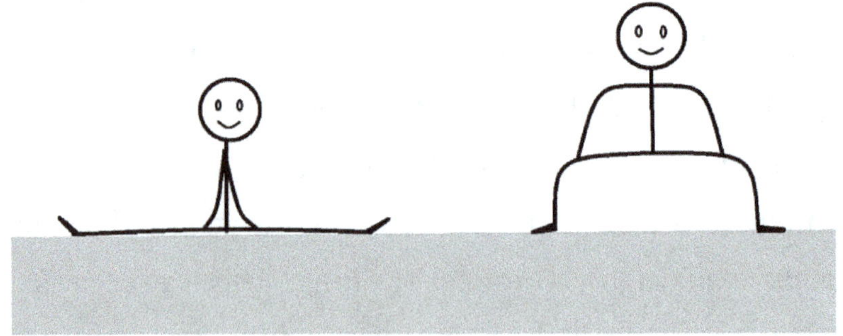

Pressure-Based Exercises: Any exercise that places pressure on the abdomen, especially when standing or sitting, can mimic the effect of straining during bowel movements. This increases intra-abdominal pressure, slows circulation in the lower abdomen, and can even contribute to the development of hemorrhoids or varicocele. When doing strength or resistance exercises, it is essential to engage the pelvic floor muscles and consider doing them in less pressurized positions like lying on your back, side, or even on all fours. This can help you avoid pushing your organs downward.

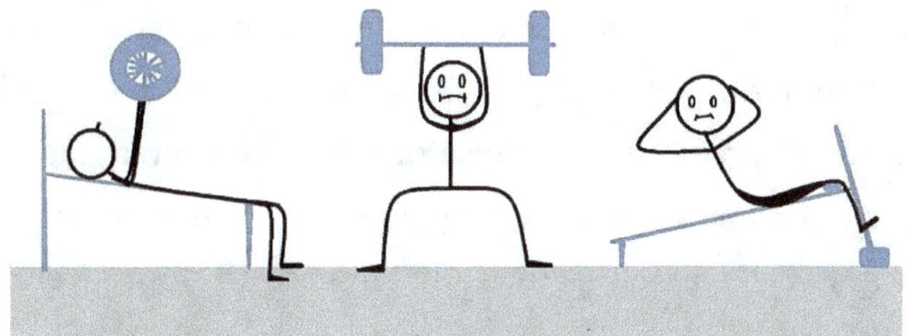

Activities to Approach with Caution

Cycling and Horse Riding: Extended periods of time on a bike or horseback can exert constant pressure on the pelvic region. This can weaken the pelvic floor if not managed carefully. To prevent issues, choose a bicycle seat that offers proper support without being too hard or narrow. It is also a good idea to take frequent breaks—about every 30 minutes— to do a few pelvic floor contractions (TCC☑) and switch to a reverse body position. This allows your pelvic muscles to recover and ensures that blood flow to the area is restored.

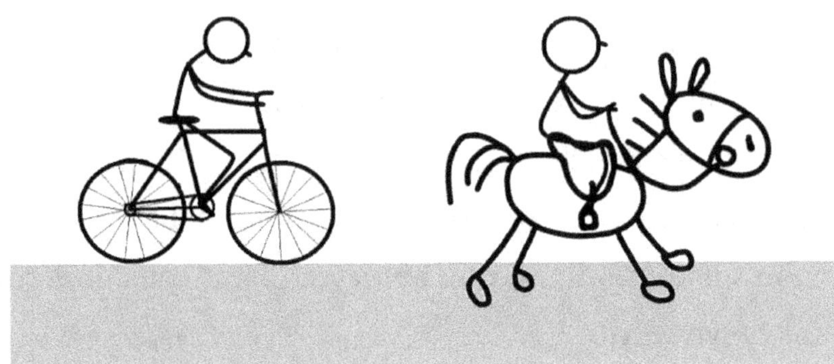

Proper Post-Exercise Care: Remember, your pelvic floor is the foundation of your core (i.e. all the muscles of the abdominal area but also those of the lumbar area and the pelvis), taking care of it will only enhance your fitness journey. By making a few adjustments to your exercise routine and being mindful of your body's signals, you can protect your pelvic health while staying active and fit.

Personal Hygiene and Bathroom Habits: Small Changes for Big Benefits

The way you take care of your body, particularly the bathroom habits, has a direct impact on your pelvic health. Many men unknowingly strain their pelvic muscles simply by rushing through these daily routines. Let's take a look at some of the best practices to protect your pelvic floor.

Best Practices for Urinary Tract Health

To preserve the intimate health and avoid urinary problems, it is worth following these key practices:

One of the simplest ways to protect the bladder and pelvic floor is through **good hygiene.** Always wash your hands before and after using the toilet. It may seem like a trivial action, but many cases of cystitis (urinary tract infections) are caused by bacteria transferred from unwashed hands. Clean hands reduce the risk of infections that can affect your bladder and prostate.

Another important factor is not holding the urine for too long. **Urinate when you feel the need!** When you feel the urge to urinate, try to go to the restroom as soon as possible. Holding urine puts unnecessary strain on the bladder and pelvic floor muscles. **Don't rush or strain!** Avoid "pushing" while urinating, as this can weaken the pelvic muscles over time. Instead, let your bladder empty naturally by relaxing the pelvic floor and abdominal muscles. When you urinate, relax and breathe normally, let the urine flow naturally without applying abdominal pressure. Try to empty your bladder completely by being patient and allowing the urine to fully exit. **Urine Leakage After Urination...A common problem among men, which can be embarrassing and often noticeable by others.** Experiencing a few drops of urine leakage after you've finished urinating is a common issue for men of all ages. Even after shaking the penis or waiting a few seconds, some urine may still leak out. This typically happens when the urethra - a 15-20 cm long tube in men, that carries urine from the bladder - doesn't empty completely, leaving a small amount of urine behind. After each urination, gently squeeze the pelvic floor muscles a few times to expel any remaining drops of urine. Another effective method is to pull back the foreskin (if applicable) and use a piece of folded toilet paper to dry the glans (head) of the penis. Then, starting at the base of the penis, gently move your fingers forward toward the tip, applying light pressure. This action will help push any trapped urine along the urethra and out of the penis. After this, perform a few more quick pelvic floor contractions, shake any remaining drops, and use toilet paper to absorb them. This reduces the risk of post-urination leakage, which can lead to irritation or infection if ignored. Finally, always wash your hands after using the toilet to maintain good hygiene.

If you experience stress-incontinence (leakage of urine when sneezing, coughing, or laughing), even your choice of footwear can make a difference. Wearing stiff-soled footwear can alter your posture and put additional pressure on your pelvic organs, potentially worsening symptoms. Opt for comfortable, supportive shoes to reduce unnecessary strain.

Protecting Your Spine: Maintaining the health of your lumbar spine is essential for urinary continence and erectile function. A strong and flexible spine supports overall pelvic health, so take care to avoid back strain and practice good posture.

By incorporating these simple habits into your daily routine, you can significantly reduce the risk of urinary issues and maintain optimal bladder and pelvic floor health.

Best Practices for Regular Bowel Movements

Taking care of rectal health with simple and mindful habits can have a significant impact on the pelvic floor. Defection is a daily function that plays a crucial role in pelvic floor health, so it's important to pay attention to how and when you go to the bathroom.

Start the day right: Begin with a calm morning routine. A peaceful and relaxed breakfast, along with a cup of warm beverage, helps stimulate the digestive system. A natural reflex called the gastrocolic reflex encourages healthy and natural bowel movement after eating, so taking time for breakfast can promote regularity. Skipping breakfast or grabbing just a quick coffee can disrupt this process, leading to irregular bowel movements. Regular meals help maintain balanced digestion and make bowel movement easier.

Fiber and Hydration: Incorporating enough fiber into your diet and staying hydrated are essential for preventing constipation and maintaining regular bowel movements. Soft and easy-to-pass stools put much less pressure on the pelvic muscles compared to hard and dry ones, so be sure to drink plenty of fluids and consume fiber-rich foods to keep the digestive system running smoothly. Increasing fiber intake without sufficient hydration can worsen constipation. Some foods, like oats for instance, absorb several times their weight in water, so it's crucial to drink more liquids when increasing fiber intake. Gradually introducing fiber-rich foods is also important to avoid bloating and trapping gas.

Don't ignore the urge: Listen to your body's signals. If you feel the urge to go to the bathroom, don't hold it in. The urge to defecate signals that the rectum is full and needs to empty. It's crucial to respond to this signal promptly rather than delay it until the sensation weakens. Postponing bowel movements can lead to constipation and unnecessary straining, which weakens the pelvic floor muscles over time. While circumstances sometimes prevent immediate restroom visits, constantly delaying bowel movements can cause the rectum to stretch over time, leading to problems like rectocele (rectal prolapse). It's essential to listen to your body and try to develop a morning routine that includes dedicated bathroom time. Even if it means setting the alarm a bit earlier, give yourself time in the morning for a calm and unrushed bathroom routine.

Regular and Proper Defecation: Regular bowel movements are crucial to overall health. Chronic constipation causes the rectum to become overly full, stretching the rectal walls. This puts pressure on the prostate and can compromise its blood circulation. To avoid straining during defecation, ensure your stool is of normal consistency by drinking enough fluids. Some men, especially those dealing with urinary incontinence, try to limit their fluid intake. However, this is a mistake. Reducing water intake can lead to dehydration, which not only worsens constipation but also causes fatigue, and may lead to headaches.

! Those men who suffer regularly from constipation get more frequently prostate inflammation, compared to the rest of the male population.

Correct posture during defecation: Your posture on the toilet is also important. Avoid slouching while sitting on the toilet, as this compresses the intestines and makes the body's natural function more difficult. Pushing with too much abdominal pressure during defecation can lead to hemorrhoids or to varicocele. Instead, focus on using minimal abdominal pressure. Straining stretches the pelvic floor muscles and ligaments, its effect is similar to lifting heavy weights regularly, which weakens the pelvic floor over time. Straining is one of the primary causes of pelvic floor dysfunction, including hemorrhoids. Maintain regular breathing and let your body do most of the work. If constipation occurs, try moving the stool by first tightening the pelvic muscles (as if you're holding back gas), then gently pressing for a short period. If straining is unavoidable, lean slightly forward, resting your elbows on your knees to avoid downward pressure on the internal organs. This position shifts the weight of the organs onto the abdominal wall instead of the pelvic floor.

Hygiene After Defecation: After defecation, it's a good habit to wash the genital area to prevent infections. If you can't wash your bottom right away, keep some wet wipes handy for convenience. Avoid using rough toilet paper, as it can irritate the sensitive skin around the anus. Also, remember to use a separate towel to dry the genital area, further reducing the risk of infections.

Protecting Perineal Veins After Defecation: Lastly, take care of the pelvic muscles after bowel movements by doing some light anal contractions to restore normal blood flow. If possible, bend forward as if you're trying to touch your ankles. This position, with your pelvis higher than your heart, helps circulation by allowing deoxygenated blood from the veins in the perineum to leave the pelvic area and be replaced by fresh, oxygen-rich blood to nourish the perineal tissues. This can relieve tension in the pelvic muscles and promote venous circulation.

Cold Water Therapy to Improve Blood Flow: To further improve blood circulation in the pelvic region, end your daily shower or bath by rinsing the genital area with cold water. Run cold water from the pubic bone to the tailbone with quick motions. After the warm shower water has dilated the blood vessels, the cold rinse makes them contract, enhancing blood flow to the lower abdomen and perineal tissues. This practice of "vascular fitness" improves the delivery of nutrients to the pelvic floor muscles, helping them stay healthy and functional.

By following these practical tips, you can maintain a healthy pelvic floor, prevent complications, and support long-term vitality and well-being.

Weight and Posture

Carrying excess weight is another common contributor to pelvic floor dysfunction. Extra body weight increases pressure on the muscles that support the bladder, the prostate and rectum. Even a modest reduction in weight can lead to significant improvements in symptoms like incontinence. Additionally, excess fat around the organs can disrupt hormone production, further influencing pelvic health. Maintaining a healthy weight is not just about appearance; it is essential for giving the body the support it needs to function optimally. Encouragingly, even small changes in weight can reduce strain on the pelvic floor muscles.

Proper posture is equally important for bladder and prostate health. Whether sitting or standing, maintaining a strong, aligned posture helps prevent unnecessary pressure on the pelvic organs. Ideally, your spine should be straight, your head lifted, and your abdomen engaged, with the pelvis tilting naturally at about a 55–65-degree angle. Poor posture—such as slumping forward with the pelvis excessively tilted—can place undue strain on the abdominal and pelvic muscles, weakening them over time.

Protect Your Bladder When Sitting and Rising

Sitting for extended periods, particularly with poor posture, compresses the pelvic floor and reduces blood flow to the area. It is essential to remain mindful of how you sit and rise, especially if your bladder is full. Rising abruptly when the bladder is full places excessive pressure on the pelvic muscles and ligaments, which over time can weaken them and lead to bladder leakage. Make it a habit to sit with a straight spine and both feet flat on the floor to maintain proper alignment and muscle support.

The Rules of Male Intimate Hygiene

When discussing male hygiene, it's important to acknowledge its impact not only on personal health but also on the health of sexual partners. Many women experience recurrent vaginal infections, often linked to male hygiene practices. While a woman may be diligent in her care, she can still face "ping-pong" infections, where bacteria transfer back and forth between partners. Since the vagina is an internal organ with a unique environment, infections can be harder to detect and treat, exacerbating this issue.

On the male side, while the urethra is farther from the anus than in women, making some infections less common, hygiene is still crucial. Poor hygiene can lead to infections that affect both partners, disrupting the harmony of sexual relationships.

How to Keep Your Penis Clean – Preventing Unpleasant Odors

Neglecting proper care of the penis can lead to infections and unpleasant odors, both of which can affect sexual health. Regular washing is essential, especially before and after sexual activity or masturbation.

- **If Circumcised**: Simply wash the penis with warm water while showering or bathing, and ensure it is thoroughly dried afterward.

- **If Uncircumcised**: Gently pull back the foreskin to clean beneath it. Do not force the foreskin further than is comfortable. Wash the head of the penis (glans) and the area under the foreskin, then pull the foreskin back in place.

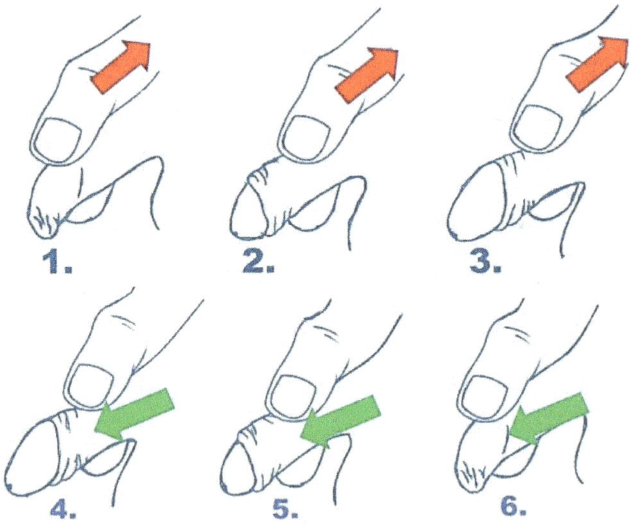

Moreover, remember to use a separate towel for drying your genital area after washing to further reduce the risk of infections.

Smegma, a natural secretion under the foreskin, helps with lubrication. However, if not cleaned regularly, it can build up, creating a breeding ground for bacteria. In uncircumcised men, smegma accumulates faster, making proper cleaning especially important. If ignored, it can lead to painful infections and, over time, may cause chronic inflammation in the prostate or other parts through the urethra. Proper hygiene of the glans can significantly reduce the risk of male urethral infections.

Studies show that women value a man's personal hygiene more than the size of his penis.

Avoid Overwashing and Irritation

While regular cleaning is important, over-washing, especially with harsh soaps, can cause irritation. Use pH-neutral shower gels designed for intimate care, avoiding aggressive soaps that may strip the protective layer on the penis. This layer helps resist infections.

Don't forget to clean the base of the penis, the testicles, and the area between the testicles and the anus. Sweat and hair can accumulate here, causing strong odors if not properly cleaned. It's also important to check your testicles monthly for any irregularities after a warm bath or shower.

Tight pants and synthetic underwear can create a warm, moist environment where bacteria thrive, so it's recommended to wear loose, cotton underwear. Regular toilet disinfection is also essential for maintaining hygiene.

The Risk of HPV Transmission

Many men carry the **HPV virus (Human Papilloma Virus)** without showing symptoms, but they can still pass it to their sexual partners. While men may remain asymptomatic, women are at higher risk due to the virus's ability to infect the deeper layers of cervical tissue, which can lead to conditions like cervical cancer.

If a man's partner is undergoing treatment for HPV-related conditions, such as cervical cancer, it's advisable for him to get tested for the virus. This reduces the risk of reinfection for his partner, whether vaginal or oral sex is involved.

Conclusion: Small Changes, Big Impact

By paying attention to the lifestyle habits—from diet and exercise to posture and sleep—you can protect and strengthen your pelvic floor for the long term. Each small adjustment can have a significant impact on these critical muscles, ensuring a lifetime of pelvic health and intimate wellness.

Chapter 5: Self-Examination

Your pelvic health is a core aspect of your overall well-being, and getting familiar with your own body is the first step toward protecting it. Have you ever wondered why this vital part of yourself is usually only examined by your andrologist or partner? By conducting a simple self-examination, you can catch early signs of changes and take proactive steps, such as pelvic floor exercises, to restore balance and strength. The truth is, we can only care for what we understand. Self-examination of the testicles is crucial for men's health, just as breast or vaginal self-exams are for women. Regular self-exams allow men to detect abnormalities early, making treatment more effective and preventing serious issues like advanced tumors or the potential removal of one or both testicles (orchiectomy).

When to Perform the Self-Examination
Taking the time to examine yourself is simple and important. Men should check their perineal area at least once a month, ideally during or after a warm bath or shower when the scrotum is relaxed, making the testicles more visible and easier to palpate.

Why It Matters

The testicles are essential to the male reproductive system. These egg-shaped organs are housed in the scrotum (sac'), which is divided into two parts by the scrotal septum, each containing one testicle. The testicles have two main functions: sperm production (spermatogenesis) and testosterone production. Testosterone is responsible for masculine characteristics like muscle mass, bone density, libido, and sexual function. A lack of testosterone can negatively affect all these areas.

How to Perform Testicular Self-Examination

The goal of testicular self-examination is to identify any unusual lumps, bumps, or growths that could signal a health issue.

1. **Warm Up:** Take a warm shower or bath first, as heat relaxes the scrotum and makes the testicles easier to examine.

2. **Visual Check:** Stand in front of a mirror to check for any visible lumps, swelling, or changes in the scrotum.

3. **Weigh Them:** Gently cradle both testicles in your palm to feel their weight. Compare the two: It's normal for one to be slightly larger or hang lower than the other. However, a sudden change in size or shape may be a red flag.

4. **Examine Each Testicle:** Using both hands, examine each testicle separately. Place your forefinger and middle finger underneath the testicle, with your thumb on top. Gently roll the testicle between your fingers, feeling for any lumps or abnormalities. Be mindful of the epididymis, a soft, coiled structure on the backside of each testicle—don't mistake it for a lump.

5. **Check for Lumps:** Suspicious lumps usually form on the sides of the testicle. They can be small (pea-sized) or larger. If you detect any abnormal growth, consult a urologist or andrologist immediately.

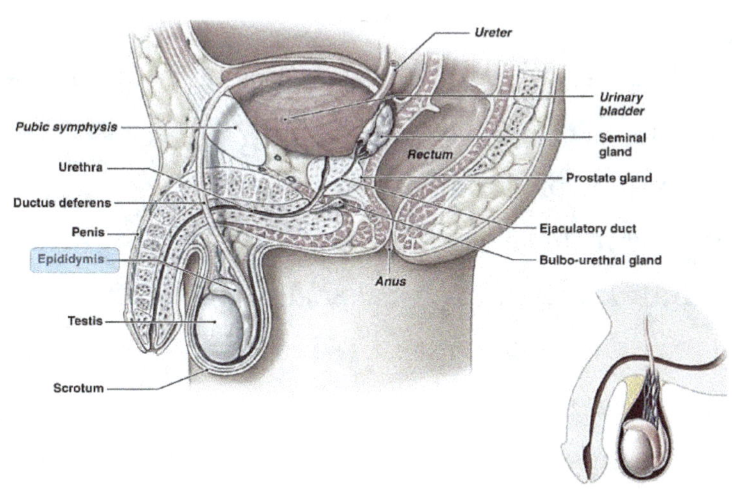

Varicocele Awareness

Varicocele is the enlargement of veins within the scrotum, typically on the left side. Minor varicoceles might go unnoticed, but larger ones can cause discomfort or dull pain, especially after prolonged standing or physical activity. This condition can negatively affect sperm production and testicular function by disrupting blood flow and raising scrotal temperature. Surgery is often required to restore normal circulation and improve fertility.

Important Note

While self-examination is valuable, it should never replace regular check-ups with a healthcare professional.

Anal Self- Check

As part of your self-exam, take a moment to check the strength of your anal sphincter, particularly if you notice any changes in bowel habits or discomfort.

How to Perform the Anal Sphincter Check: Using your fingertip, gently touch the external anal sphincter. It should feel firm and closed without squeezing. When you intentionally squeeze the muscle around the anus, it should tighten significantly. You can also use a mirror to visually inspect the area for any bulges, tenderness, or bleeding.

Signs of Weakness: Early signs of sphincter weakness include difficulty holding back gas, particularly during activities that increase intra-abdominal pressure, such as standing up, laughing, or coughing. In more severe cases, you may notice soiling of underwear, difficulty with bowel movements, or even fecal incontinence.

If you experience rectal bleeding, it is important to consult a healthcare provider, as the cause can only be diagnosed through a proper medical exam (visit a proctologist).

Impact of Constipation and Rectal Health

Chronic constipation not only increases the risk of rectal issues but is also linked to a higher incidence of prostate inflammation. The rectum is designed to expand to accommodate fecal matter, but delaying bowel movements repeatedly can overstretch these tissues, leading to complications like rectal prolapse or hemorrhoids.

After exploring the anal sphincter do not touch the "head" or the "tip" of the penis (called glans) since through the urethral opening you can 'send' some bacteria up causing urinary tract infection! Hygiene is key to staying healthy!

Hemorrhoids as Lifestyle Adaptation

Hemorrhoidal plexuses are part of the normal human anatomy of the anal canal. They should not be considered pathological. These arteriovenous pads are covered with a mucous membrane and function to ensure a hermetic closure for the anus in all three dimensions. They become pathological when lengthened, swollen, or inflamed and protruding outside through the anus.

Individuals suffering from hemorrhoids may experience varying degrees of discomfort. This condition often stems from lifestyle choices—prolonged sitting, straining during bowel movements, or heavy lifting can all contribute to the problem. The body adjusts to these bad habits, and over time, if left untreated, it can lead to significant discomfort, itching, and bleeding.

Key Takeaway

Maintaining healthy bowel habits and avoiding unnecessary strain is crucial for protecting the health of your perineal tissues and preventing complications like hemorrhoids or rectal prolapse.

Caring for Your Body Means Understanding It

Self-exams help you stay in touch with your body's changes and give you the confidence to address any issues early. Many conditions, like stress incontinence, prostatitis, and rectocele, can develop over time due to poor lifestyle habits, like straining during bowel movements, slouching, or skipping pelvic floor exercises. When we neglect these muscles, the organs they support—like the bladder, prostate and rectum—may begin to shift, causing discomfort and functional problems.

Whether you have just started pelvic floor exercises or have been practicing them for a while, your self-exam will serve as a guide to monitor your progress. Embrace the process as a vital part of self-care. Your body, especially the parts men often ignore, deserves your attention.

A Final Word

One of the greatest benefits of Kegel exercises is their adaptability—you can tailor them to suit your unique needs and goals at any stage of life. Like any fitness routine, it is important to personalize your Kegel exercises. For example, if your goal is to prevent or manage incontinence, you may want to focus on a mix of strengthening exercises that involve both fast and slow contractions. On the other hand, if sexual health is your priority, incorporating relaxation techniques into your Kegel routine can enhance blood flow and sensitivity. Regardless of your focus, consistency is essential. Aim for at least 10 minutes of exercise a day or three sessions a week to build and maintain strong pelvic floor muscles.

This is a lifelong practice, much like brushing your teeth, and it should become a part of your daily routine. Keep in mind that if you stop doing the exercises, your muscles will weaken over time. The secret to lasting results is regular practice, and the IWT® program you have learned about is an excellent way to stay on track.

While you may experience ups and downs along the way, remember that pelvic floor health is a journey, not a race. It's normal to face challenges, but with the right mindset, the proper tools, and a holistic approach, you'll be well on your way to achieving lifelong intimate health and confidence.

I have shared practical advice throughout this book to help you integrate these exercises into your life starting today. Treat your body as a valuable asset, one worth protecting and nurturing for the long run. Ultimately, your health and well-being are in your hands, and the work you put into caring for your pelvic floor will pay off in many ways.

Congratulations on taking this important step toward better sexual health and pelvic floor strength. Stay consistent, be patient, and prioritize your well-being—you deserve it!

Congratulations on starting your journey toward better sexual health!

Glossary

Anal Sphincters: Two rings of muscles surrounding the rectum and anus that help control the passage of bowel movements.

Anus: The final two inches of the rectum, surrounded by the internal and external anal sphincter muscles, serving as the outlet for solid waste (stool).

Bacteria: Microscopic, one-celled organisms. Some bacteria are harmless or beneficial, while others can cause infections. Most prostate infections are caused by common bacteria found in the gastrointestinal system.

Benign Prostatic Hyperplasia (BPH): A condition characterized by the non-cancerous enlargement of the prostate gland, often resulting in voiding difficulties.

Bladder: A stretchable, muscular organ located inside the pelvic cavity that retains urine until it is excreted from the body; supported by the pelvic floor muscles.

Bowel Movement: The act of passing feces (stool) through the anus.

Bowels: Another term for the intestines or colon.

Bulbocavernosus Muscle: In males, this muscle encircles the bulb or root of the penis and connects it to the perineal body. It plays a crucial role in voluntary urination and helps empty the urethra at the end of urination, as well as expels semen during ejaculation.

Calculus: A hardened, stonelike mass of high calcium content that can form in the kidneys, bladder, or prostate. Prostate stones are generally not dangerous but may negatively influence normal function and contribute to chronic prostatitis or, in some cases, prostate cancer.

Catheter: A narrow, flexible tube inserted into the urethra and bladder for the purpose of draining urine.

Chronic Prostatitis: A persistent form of prostatitis that can last for an extended period—sometimes years.

Colon: The lower section of the large intestine leading into the rectum.

Constipation: A condition characterized by infrequent, hard, dry bowel movements that are difficult and uncomfortable to evacuate.

Continence: The ability to exercise voluntary control over the urge to urinate or defecate until an appropriate time and place.

Contraindication: A medical condition or factor that makes a particular treatment or procedure inadvisable due to increased risk.

Cystitis: Inflammation of the bladder, usually caused by an infection.

Cystoscopy: A diagnostic procedure that allows direct visualization of the urethra and bladder using a specialized instrument.

Defecate: The act of having a bowel movement.

Dehydration: A state that occurs when the body loses more fluid than it takes in, leading to insufficient hydration.

Diuretic: Any drug, beverage, or food that promotes increased urine production and excretion.

Ejaculation: The ejection of sperm and seminal fluid from the penis, resulting from the contraction of muscles in the urethra and prostate area.

Epididymis: A coiled tube located at the back of each testicle that stores and matures sperm.

Estrogen: A key female sex hormone that regulates sexual development and function, contributing to the development of female sex characteristics. In men, the amount of estrogen secreted by the testicles is particularly modest, although biologically important.

Evacuation: Another term for a bowel movement.

External Sphincter: The outer layer of the sphincter muscle, usually under voluntary control, helping to regulate bowel and urinary functions.

Fecal Incontinence: The accidental and involuntary loss of fecal material (stool) or gas from the anus.

Feces (Stool): Waste material produced from the intestines, composed of bacteria, undigested food, and other materials.

Flatulence: The release of gas through the anus, often resulting from digestion.

Fungal Infection: An infection caused by fungi, such as Candida, which can affect various body parts, including the prostate.

Gas: Material produced from swallowed air, certain foods, or the breakdown of waste material by bacteria in the colon.

Impotence: The inability of a man to achieve or maintain an erection sufficient for satisfactory sexual performance.

Incontinence: The inability to retain urine within the bladder or feces within the colon, which can be complete or partial.

Internal Sphincter: The internal layer of the sphincter muscle, usually under involuntary control.

Intra-abdominal: Located within the abdominal cavity.

Kegel Exercises: Exercises involving the repetitive contraction of the pelvic floor muscles, aimed at strengthening these muscles to decrease or eliminate incontinence and other intimate issues.

Kidneys: Two glandular organs that filter blood to remove waste products and excess substances, producing urine.

Levator Ani: The main muscle of the pelvic floor, composed of several parts that support pelvic organs.

Lower Back Pain: Discomfort in the lower back region, which may frequently arise from prostate disorders.

Magnesium: An essential metallic mineral that may play a significant role in prostate health.

Orchiectomy: Surgical removal of one or both testicles.

Overflow Incontinence: The involuntary loss of urine associated with an overdistended bladder.

Pelvic Floor: The muscle structure at the base of the abdominal cavity that supports the pelvic organs.

Pelvic Floor Muscles: A group of muscles below the pelvic organs that assist in maintaining continence.

Pelvic Organ Prolapse: A condition in which one or more pelvic organs descend from their normal position, potentially leading to various symptoms.

Penis: The male organ used for urination and sexual intercourse.

Perineum: The area of muscle and tissue located between the scrotum and anus.

Premature Ejaculation: A male sexual dysfunction in which ejaculation occurs before the desired time, potentially impacting sexual satisfaction for both partners.

Prostate: A firm, muscular gland in males that surrounds the urethra and plays a key role in reproductive health.

Prostate Massage: A technique involving the stimulation of the prostate through the rectum, often used to relieve congestion or obtain samples for testing.

Prostatectomy: Surgical removal of all or part of the prostate gland, typically to treat prostate cancer.

Prostatitis: Inflammation or infection of the prostate, which can be acute or chronic.

Pubic Bone: The lower front part of the pelvis.

Pubic Symphysis: The joint where the two pubic bones meet.

Pubococcygeus (PC) Muscle: The muscle group that supports the pelvic organs; Kegel exercises are designed to strengthen these muscles.

Pudendal Nerves: Nerves that innervate the external urethral and anal sphincters and the pelvic and urogenital diaphragm muscles, part of the voluntary nervous system.

Radical Prostatectomy: The complete surgical removal of the prostate gland to treat prostate cancer.

Rectocele: A condition in which the anterior or posterior rectal wall bulges into the vagina, more common in women.

Rectum: The final section of the intestines, connecting to the anus.

Reflex Incontinence: Involuntary loss of urine due to overactivity of the bladder muscle, without the sensation of urgency.

Risk Factor: A characteristic or condition that increases an individual's likelihood of developing a specific disease.

Scrotum: The external pouch of skin that contains and protects the testicles and epididymis.

Sphincter: A group of circular muscles surrounding an opening in the body, controlling the flow of fluids through the opening.

Stress Incontinence: A type of urinary incontinence characterized by involuntary leakage of urine during physical activities that increase abdominal pressure, such as coughing, sneezing, or exercising.

Testicles: Two glands located in the scrotum that produce sperm and testosterone.

Testosterone: The principal male sex hormone responsible for male sexual characteristics and the growth of prostatic tissue.

Urethra: A muscular tube connecting the bladder to the outside, responsible for carrying urine away from the bladder.

Urge Incontinence: A form of urinary incontinence characterized by sudden, involuntary leakage of urine when the bladder muscle contracts unexpectedly.

Urinary Incontinence: The loss of control over urinary storage function, leading to involuntary leakage of urine.

Urinary Retention: A condition in which urine backs up in the bladder, potentially leading to bladder and kidney damage.

Urologist: A physician specializing in disorders of the urinary system and male reproductive organs.

Vaginal Yeast Infection: An infection in women caused by yeast organisms, which can be sexually transmitted and may also lead to prostatitis.

Voluntary Control: Conscious, intentional control over bodily functions.

Zinc: An essential metallic mineral important for various bodily functions, including prostate health; the prostate contains a high concentration of zinc.

# # #

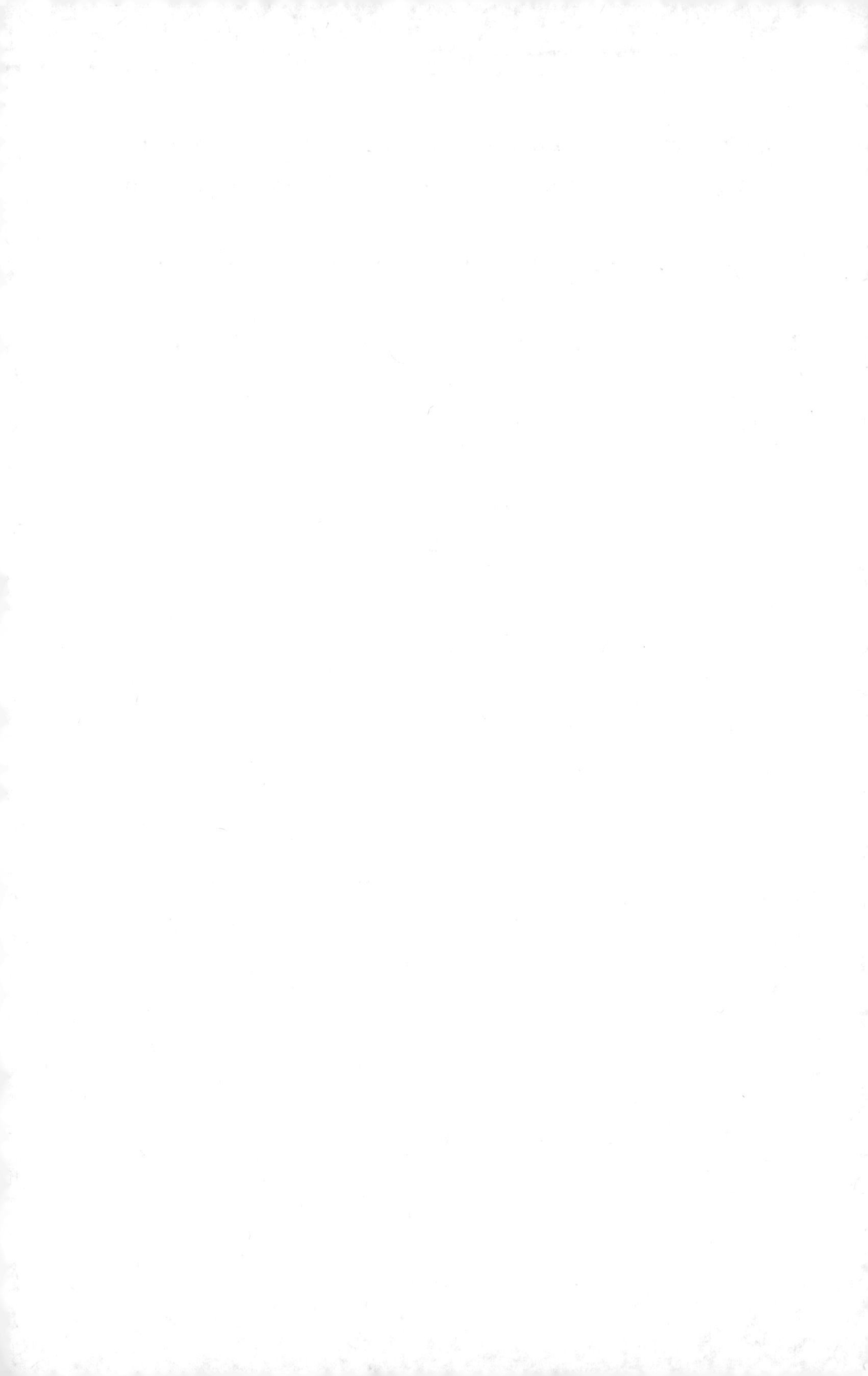